Gluten Free Snacks, Desserts, Treats and Breakfast Ideas

The Easy Gluten-Free Cookbook

Table of Contents

Gluten Free Breakfast Recipes

Cowboy Breakfast Skillet

Creole Frittata

Coconut and Banana Pancakes

Pumpkin & Bacon Pancakes

Tapioca Blueberry Crepes

Cashew Belgian Waffles

Apple Upside Down Cakes

Chicken Breakfast Patties

Crunchy Grain-Free Granola

Carrot Cake Pancakes

Bacon and Sweet Potato Hash

Apple and Pulled Pork Hash Cakes

Ham, Egg & Veggie Breakfast Burrito

GF Breakfast Pizza

Turkey Bacon Club Salad

GF Cobb Salad

GF Crab Cakes

No-Oats Oatmeal

Acorn Squash 'N Eggs
Beef and Plantain Stir-Fry
GF Tuna Spread
GF Egg In A Hole
GF Apple Nut Bake
Bacon & Fruit Scramble
Salmon & Veggie Breakfast Salad

Kids Lunch Recipes
Pita Bites
Homemade Applesauce
Banana Pudding
Pizza Bites
Soft Baked Pretzel
Frontier Anzac Biscuits
Cream Filled Carrot Cake Muffin
Sausage Stuffed "Corn" Muffin
Baby BLT
Cheese Steak Sandwich
Cashew Butter and Banana Sandwich
Almond Butter and Strawberry Sandwich
Beef Bun
Cocoa Cream Bun

Honey Nut Bun
Chicken Pot Pie
Lamb Pot Pie
My Favorite Meatballs
Bacon Baked Apples
Peach Pecan "Fried" Pie
Sweet Potato "Fried" Pie
Asian Empanada
Jamaican Jerk Patty
Chicken Tenders
Turkey Tenders

Snack Recipes
Gluten-Free Snack Introduction
Spicy Chicken Bites
Highland Scotch Egg
Jalapeño Bacon Bites
Fried Green Tomatoes
Bacon Mofongo
Guilt-Free Guacamole
Coconut Shrimp
Green Deviled Eggs 'N Ham
Piggies in a Poke

Mighty Beef Sliders

Zucchini Rollatini

Bacon Quesadilla

Chicken Taquitos

Sausage And Peppers

Baked Sweet Plantains

Ants On A Log

Grilled Pineapple Fruit Salad

Sweet Cinnamon Gluten-Free Pretzel

Blueberry Dumplings

Sweet Papaya Fried Pie

Fried Choco Pie

Chocolate Banana Bites

Fruit 'N Nut Bars

Hoppin' Hot Chocolate

Piña Colada Smoothie

Gluten-Free Snack Conclusion

Bread Recipes

"Corn" Muffins

Gluten-Free English Muffins

Skillet Biscuits
Italian Flatbread
Indian Naan
State Fair Fry Bread
Easy Pocket Pita
Frontier Tortillas
Coconut Crisps
Strawberry Bread
Primal Apple Cider Bread
Pumpkin Coconut Bread
Avocado Spice Bread
Cocoa Bread
Grain-Free Gingerbread
Citrus Curry Spice Bread
Banana Nut Bread
Simple Squash Muffins
Sunshine Muffins
Cranberry Pistachio Scones
Sweet Potato Basil Rolls
Garlic 'N Herb Rolls
Savory Tomato Rolls
Sage Sausage Buns
New Yorkshire Puddings

Baking Recipes

Coconut Macaroons

Blackberry Dumplings
Carrot Cake Cookie Bars
Golden Coconut Cake
Chocolate Zucchini Cake
Apple Turnover Pastries
Cocoa Cream Muffins
Ginger Spice Cookies
Lemon Coconut Bars
Sweet Potato Cinnamon Rolls
Candied Banana Bread
Orange Cranberry Muffins
Mocha Brownie Bites
Blueberry Scones
Double Pumpkin Muffins
Cinnamon Raisin Bread
Sandwich Rolls
Bagels
All-Purpose Pizza Crust
Perfectly Pita
Sesame Pretzel Sticks
Breakfast Buns

Avocado Club Muffin
Chicken Dumpling Bun
Lemon Poppy Seed Muffins

Gluten Free Breakfast Recipes

Cowboy Breakfast Skillet

Prep Time: 5 minutes

Cook Time: 15 minutes

Servings: 2

The first thing that comes to mind when I read the name Cowboy Breakfast Skillet is a question. Does it come with a cowboy? Sorry ladies, no fella but it does come with a good dose of delicious protein to start your day off right. Protein is an important part of your recommended daily dietary requirements, but getting enough can be tricky. Eating food like the Cowboy Breakfast Skillet will ensure that your body gets what it needs to stay strong and healthy. Eat well and be ready. You never know when you might need to jump on a horse and ride off into the sunset.

INGREDIENTS

6 cage-free eggs

8 oz ground pork sausage

1 medium sweet potato

1 bell pepper

1 small red onion

Ground black pepper, to taste

Paprika, to taste

Celtic sea salt, to taste

Pinch of cinnamon (optional)

INSTRUCTIONS

1. Bring medium pot to boil with lightly salted water. Leave enough room in pot for sweet potato. Heat large skillet over medium-high heat.

2. Peel and dice sweet potato. Add to boiling water for 5 minutes.

3. Add sausage to hot skillet. Brown sausage for 5 minutes, stirring occasionally with wooden spatula.

4. While potatoes and sausage cook, seed and vein bell pepper and peel onion, then dice.

5. Beat eggs with spices in medium bowl with hand mixer or whisk.

6. Once browned, add pepper and onion to sausage. Sauté about 2 minutes, until vegetables are tender and a bit caramelized.

7. Drain sweet potatoes in colander and add to skillet. Sauté about 1 minute, until any excess liquid is evaporated. Then pour in egg mixture.

8. Scramble eggs with wooden spatula. Reduce skillet to medium heat to cook eggs evenly and avoid browning.

9. Cook and stir eggs until desired firmness. Remove from heat and serve.

Creole Frittata

Prep Time: 5 minutes

Cook Time: 15 minutes

Servings: 4

There is said to be a basic difference between Creole and Cajun cooking. A Creole feeds one family with three chickens and a Cajun feeds three families with one chicken. That be said, the Creole style of cooking originated in New Orleans, Louisiana and has held a hard and steady reputation as being one of the most flavorful styles of cooking in America. This simple Creole Frittata will set your heart to singing and it is just as good at breakfast as it is at any time of day. We guarantee you that sausage and eggs have never tasted so happy as this.

INGREDIENTS

4 Andouille sausage links

12 cage-free eggs

1 green bell pepper

1 red bell pepper

1 medium sweet onion

2 tablespoons paprika

1 teaspoon cayenne pepper

1 teaspoon onion powder

1 teaspoon garlic powder

1 teaspoon dried oregano

1 teaspoon dried thyme

1 teaspoon dried basil

1 teaspoon black pepper

1 tablespoon Celtic sea salt

Coconut oil (for cooking)

INSTRUCTIONS

1. Lightly coat large cast iron skillet with lid with coconut oil and heat over medium-high heat.
2. Cut sausage links on bias into 1/2 inch slices. Add to hot skillet.
3. While sausage browns, stem and seed peppers, and peel onion. Cut onions and peppers in half, then into 1/4 inch slices. Add to skillet and stir with wooden spatula. Sauté about 2 minutes.
4. Beat eggs with spices in large bowl with hand mixer or whisk.
5. Add eggs to browned sausage and softened veggies.
6. Reduce skillet to medium-low heat and cover with well fitting lid. Cook for about 10 minutes.
7. When eggs are firm throughout, remove from heat. Slice and serve.

Coconut and Banana Pancakes

Prep Time: 5 minutes

Cook Time: 15 minutes

Servings: 2

Calling all monkeys! Just the name Coconut and Banana Pancakes brings the islands to mind, doesn't it? Families of all sizes love to sit around the breakfast table with a big stack of flapjacks. Memories are made of moments like this. These pancakes have just enough touch of fresh coconut flavor to soak up the goodness of the sweet banana topping and start your morning off right.

INGREDIENTS

Pancakes:

1 3/4 cups almond meal

1 teaspoon baking powder

2 cage-free eggs

3/4 cup coconut milk

1/4 cup flaked coconut

1/2 banana

1 teaspoon vanilla

1/4 teaspoon Celtic sea salt

Coconut oil (for cooking)

Topping:

1/2 banana

Agave nectar (optional)

INSTRUCTIONS

1. Heat a large skillet over medium-high heat and lightly coat with coconut oil.

2. Mash 1/2 banana in medium bowl with fork. Whisk in eggs, then coconut milk and vanilla.

3. Add almond flour, salt and baking powder. Whisk until smooth. Fold in coconut flakes.

4. Use ladle or dry measure cup to pour 1/4 cup of batter onto hot oiled skillet. Fit 2 or 3 pancakes comfortably, so they do not touch as they spread.

5. Cook until sides of pancakes are firm and batter bubbles up a bit. About 3 to 4 minutes.

6. Carefully flip pancakes with spatula and cook for additional minute, or until cooked through. Repeat with remaining batter. Re-oil pan if necessary. Pancakes will be slightly delicate, so flip and plate with care.

7. Slice 1/2 banana. Top with banana slices and agave nectar. Serve warm.

Pumpkin & Bacon Pancakes

Prep Time: 5 minutes

Cook Time: 15 minutes

Servings: 2

When you're in the mood for something fun yet hearty and healthy, head for these Pumpkin & Bacon Pancakes. Bacon just makes everything better, doesn't it? Try rolling one of these around scrambled eggs, or the kids in all of us love them with a smidge of nut butter. The pumpkin in this recipe makes these pancakes nice and moist and the bacon gives them that highly desired sweet and salty taste combination.

INGREDIENTS

1 3/4 cups almond flour

1 cup almond milk

1/2 cup pumpkin puree

2 eggs

1 teaspoon baking powder

2 teaspoons ground cinnamon

1 teaspoon vanilla

1/4 teaspoon Celtic sea salt

4 slices nitrate-free bacon

INSTRUCTIONS

1. Heat large skillet over high heat.
2. Chop bacon into 1/2 inch pieces. Add to hot skillet and brown. Stir occasionally with wooden spoon.
3. Whisk eggs in medium bowl. Then whisk in almond milk, pumpkin puree, vanilla and cinnamon.
4. Add almond flour, salt and baking powder. Whisk until smooth.
5. Once crisp, reduce pan to medium heat and remove bacon from pan, leaving drippings. Drain bacon bits on paper towel, then stir into pancake mixture.
6. Use ladle or dry measure cup to pour 1/4 cup of batter onto hot oiled skillet. Fit 2 or 3 pancakes comfortably, so they do not touch as they spread.
7. Cook until sides of pancakes are firm and batter bubbles up a bit. About 3 to 4 minutes.
8. Carefully flip pancakes with spatula and cook for additional minute, or until cooked through. Repeat with remaining batter. Pancakes will be slightly delicate, so flip and plate with care.
9. Serve warm. Top with topping of choice.

Tapioca Blueberry Crepes

Prep Time: 5 minutes

Cook Time: 15 minutes

Servings: 2

How could you possibly go wrong with these fantastic crepes that are both stuffed and topped? First you have the delicate outer layer, then the warm fruity filling to bite into. Add just a touch of slightly sweet and creamy topping to every bite and you've got a family award winner for sure. The best part is, there is no better way to get a load of morning antioxidants into your tummy. This just may be a Sunday morning favorite.

INGREDIENTS

Crêpes:

1 cup tapioca flour/starch

1 cup coconut milk

1 cage-free egg

Pinch Celtic sea salt

Coconut oil (for cooking)

Filling:

1 pint blueberries

2 tablespoons sweetener*

1 teaspoon vanilla

Pinch ground black pepper

Pinch Celtic sea salt

1 tablespoon water

Topping:

1/2 cup coconut crème

2 tablespoons agave nectar

1/2 teaspoon vanilla

Coconut milk (for thinning)

INSTRUCTIONS

1. Heat large non-stick pan over medium heat. Add small dollop of coconut oil and carefully spread with wadded paper towel to coat evenly . Preserve paper towel.

2. Heat medium pan over medium heat. Add all *Filling* ingredients except water. Stir occasionally with wooden spoon. Add extra tablespoon of water if blueberries do not break down enough. Remove from heat when sufficiently warmed and saucy.

3. Combine all *Crêpe* ingredients in a medium bowl. Blend thoroughly.

4. When large non-stick pan is hot, use ladle or dry measure cup to pour in 1/3 cup of crêpe batter while tilting pan in all directions to evenly spread batter.

5. Cook crêpe about 2 minutes, then carefully flip and cook another 1 - 2 minutes.

6. When both sides are lightly browned, remove crêpe to plate and oil pan with wadded paper towel. Repeat process of cooking crêpe and oiling pan with remaining batter.

7. Blend all *Topping* ingredients. Thin with small amount of coconut milk to create drizzling consistency if necessary.

8. Fill crêpes with blueberry compote down center and fold over each side. Plate fold-side down and drizzle on coconut crème **Topping**. Serve warm.

stevia, raw honey, or agave nectar

Cashew Belgian Waffles

Prep Time: 10 minutes

Cook Time: 10 minutes

Servings: 2

It is said that King Charles IX of France ruled that waffle vendors had to set up their stalls at least 12 feet away from each other as eating waffles was so popular. Can you imagine? Those must have been some pretty big waffle eaters to require 6 foot on each side just for elbow room! These light crispy waffles have the added bonus of protein derived from cashew flour. Serve topped with warm fruit compote and you have a treat fit for a king!

INGREDIENTS

Waffles:

1 cup cashew flour (or finely ground raw cashews)

1/4 coconut flour

3 cage-free eggs, separated

1/4 cup coconut oil

4 tablespoons sweetener

1 tablespoon aluminum-free baking soda

1 teaspoon vanilla

1 pinch Celtic sea salt

1 teaspoon ground cinnamon (optional)

Topping:

1 cup fresh fruit

1/2 teaspoon vanilla

2 tablespoons water

1 tablespoon sweetener*

DIRECTIONS

1. Preheat waffle iron. Use wadded paper towel to carefully coat with coconut oil.
2. Combine flours, salt and baking soda in small bowl. In large bowl, whisk together egg yolks, oil, vanilla, plus sweetener and cinnamon (optional).
3. In separate bowl, beat egg whites to medium-stiff peaks with hand mixer. Stir flour mixture into the egg yolk mixture. Gently fold egg whites into batter.
4. Pour portion of batter onto hot waffle iron. Cook 4 - 5 minutes, until golden brown and crisp. Repeat with remain batter
5. While waffles are cooking, combine all *Topping* ingredients in small pan. Cook over stovetop until reduced and thick.
6. Top waffles with fruit compote or agave syrup (optional). Serve hot.

stevia, raw honey, or agave nectar

Apple Upside Down Cakes

Prep Time: 5 minutes

Cook Time: 15 minutes

Servings: 2

Upside down cake is always so popular—this recipe make it even better because it is for fun individually size pancakes. Each has its own portion of beautifully caramelized apples on top. If only it were easier to bake while standing on your head, we'd make them every day. Hang in there; you'll get the knack of it after a while. Kidding aside, we think you'll agree, there's no better way to get your apple a day.

INGREDIENTS

1 3/4 cups almond meal

2 cage-free eggs

3/4 cup almond milk

2 tablespoons sweetener*

1 teaspoon baking powder

Juice of 1/2 lemon

1 teaspoon vanilla

1 teaspoon ground cinnamon

1 teaspoon ground nutmeg

1/4 teaspoon salt

1 tart apple

1/2 cup crushed pecans

INSTRUCTIONS

1. Heat large skillet over medium-high heat and lightly coat with coconut oil.

2. In medium bowl combine lemon juice, vanilla, cinnamon and nutmeg.

3. Peel and core apple, then slice in half length-wise. Lay halves down on flat side and slice thinly from top of apple to bottom. Carefully toss apple slices in lemon juice and spices. Try not to break any.

4. Arrange apple slices into a circle by overlapping at the bottom and fanning out. Try to make at least 4 circles.

5. Add eggs and almond milk into leftover lemon juice and spices and whisk until combined. Add almond flour, salt and baking powder. Whisk until smooth.

6. Use oiled spatula to lift apples, keeping their arrangement, and place into hot pan. Get at least two apple arrangements into pan together. Sprinkle chopped pecans into pan around apple circles.

7. Use ladle or dry measure cup to pour 1/3 cup of batter over and around apple arrangements in skillet. Do not let pancakes touch as they spread.

8. Cook until sides of pancakes are firm and batter bubbles up a bit. About 3 - 4 minutes.

9. Flip pancakes with spatula, careful not to disturb apples. Cook for additional minute, or until cooked through. Repeat with remaining batter. Re-oil pan if necessary.

10. Pancakes will be slightly delicate, so flip and plate with care.

11. Sprinkle with cinnamon. Serve warm.

*stevia, raw honey, or agave nectar

Chicken Breakfast Patties

Prep Time: 5 minutes

Cook Time: 10 minutes

Servings: 2

It's breakfast time and it's time for that old trick question too. What came first, the chicken or the egg? Well, in this case the chicken wins and so do you with these delicious Chicken Breakfast Patties. It's alright if you decide to make it fair and serve them alongside a couple of sunny-side up eggs. This dish gives you a protein power punch and fires up your energy engine for a nice productive day.

INGREDIENTS

8 oz chicken

1 cage-free egg

1/4 cup coconut flour

1/2 sweet onion

1 tablespoon apple cider vinegar

1 teaspoon ground black pepper

1 teaspoon Celtic sea salt

1 teaspoon paprika

1 teaspoon ground sage

1 teaspoon dried thyme

1 teaspoon fennel seed (optional)

1/2 teaspoon nutmeg (optional)

1 tablespoon water

Coconut oil (for cooking)

INSTRUCTIONS

1. Heat medium skillet over medium heat and lightly coat with coconut oil.

2. Grind chicken meat and peeled 1/2 onion to medium grind in food processor, bullet blender, or meat grinder. Or grind onion alone and add to pre-ground chicken in medium bowl.

3. Add apple cider vinegar, spices and 1 tablespoon coconut flour to ground chicken and onion. Mix well until combined. Form into 2 large or 4 small patties and place on plate.

4. Beat egg with water and pour egg wash over patties. Gently flip patties to get them evenly covered with egg wash. Take coconut flour and sprinkle over both sides of egg washed patties. Pat coconut flour gently into patties.

5. Place coated patties into hot oiled skillet and cook about 3 - 4 minutes, until golden brown and crisp. Flip and cook another 3 - 4 minutes, or until done.

6. Remove cooked patties from pan and drain on paper towel. Serve hot.

Crunchy Grain-Free Granola

Prep Time: 5 minutes

Cook Time: 20 minutes

Servings: 4

"Grain free granola?" you say. Yep, you read it right! This medley of fruits and nuts mixed with the warm spiciness of cinnamon and nutmeg can't be beat. One mouthful and nobody is going to miss any grains. Our recipe for Grain Free Granola is a great one to make in a double batch. Have some now, and pack up extra treat size packs for special lunchbox or desk drawer treats.

INGREDIENTS

1 cup almond flour

1/4 cup ground chia seed (or flax seed meal)

1 tablespoon vanilla

1 teaspoon ground nutmeg

1 teaspoon ground cinnamon

1/2 cup raw agave nectar (or 1/2 cup raw honey + 1 tablespoon water)

1 cup flaked coconut

1 cup sliced almonds

1/2 cup dried figs

1/2 cup dried dates

1/2 cup pecans

1/2 cup pumpkin seeds

1/2 cup dried apricots

1/2 cup coconut oil, melted

INSTRUCTIONS

1. Preheat oven to 350 degrees F. Lightly coat cookie sheet with coconut oil.

2. Stem figs and pit dates. Chop figs, dates, pecans and apricots. Add to medium bowl, along with all other ingredients. Mix to combine, then spread evenly over sheet pan with spatula.

3. Bake in preheated oven for about 10 minutes. Then carefully remove and use spatula to turn over par-baked granola. Bake for additional 8 - 10 minutes. Check periodically to ensure nuts do not over-toast.

4. Remove from oven and let cool and firm. Serve cool.

Carrot Cake Pancakes

Prep Time: 5 minutes

Cook Time: 15 minutes

Servings: 2

Oh yum, just the name of this recipe says it all. Remember the spicy aroma of freshly baked carrot cake? You're about to smell it again and better yet, taste it. Our version comes disguised as a stack of pancakes and is chock full of heart healthy goodness. Our recipe also ensures that you'll never find yourself looking for walnuts or raisins like a lost treasure hunt. You'll find them popping up in every bite!

INGREDIENTS

1 3/4 cups almond meal

2 cage-free eggs

3/4 cup almond milk

2 medium carrots

1/4 cup chopped walnuts

1/4 cup golden raisins (optional)

1 teaspoon baking powder

1 tablespoon ground cinnamon

1 teaspoon ground nutmeg

1 teaspoon ground ginger

1 teaspoon vanilla

1/4 teaspoon Celtic sea salt

Pinch of ground black pepper

INSTRUCTIONS

1. Heat large skillet on medium-high heat and lightly coat with oil.

2. Finely grate carrots and drain in paper towel, or roughly process in food processor or bullet blender.

3. In medium bowl whisk eggs, almond milk, vanilla, cinnamon, nutmeg, ginger and black pepper.

4. Add almond flour, salt and baking powder. Whisk until smooth. Stir in carrots, walnuts and raisins (optional).

5. Use ladle or dry measure cup to pour 1/3 cup of batter onto hot oiled skillet. Fit 2 or 3 pancakes comfortably, so they do not touch as they spread.

6. Cook until sides of pancakes are firm and batter bubbles up a bit. About 3 - 4 minutes.

7. Carefully flip pancakes with spatula and cook for additional minute, or until cooked through. Repeat with remaining batter. Re-oil pan if necessary. Pancakes will be slightly delicate, so flip and plate with care.

8. Serve warm. Sprinkle with cinnamon and drizzle with agave nectar, or topping of choice.

Bacon and Sweet Potato Hash

Prep Time: 10 minutes

Cook Time: 10 minutes

Servings: 2

Hash is one of the all-time favorite ways to use leftover potatoes with just about anything else you can pull out of your refrigerator! We've stepped that concept up and over with our version of Bacon and Sweet Potato Hash. Sweet potatoes are one of the most highly ranked vegetables on the nutritional scale which officially puts them on the list of superfoods. Our bodies crave nutrients like these, so why not make them a great part of our morning routine?

INGREDIENTS

8 oz nitrate-free bacon (thick cut slices or whole slab)

1 medium sweet potato

1 small white onion

1 teaspoon ground cinnamon

1 teaspoon dried thyme

1 teaspoon rosemary

INSTRUCTIONS

1. Bring medium pot to boil with lightly salted water. Leave enough room in pot for sweet potato. Heat a large skillet over high heat.
2. Chop bacon into 1/2 inch pieces or cubes. Add to hot skillet and brown. Stir occasionally with wooden spoon.
3. Peel and dice sweet potato. Add to boiling water for about 4 minutes, until tender but not mushy.

4. While potatoes and bacon cook, peel and dice onion.

5. Once browned, add onion to bacon. Sauté about 1 minute, until onions are tender and a bit caramelized.

6. Drain sweet potatoes in colander and add to skillet. Sprinkle on cinnamon, thyme and rosemary. Sauté 1 - 2 minutes, until any excess liquid is evaporated and everything is lightly caramelized and cooked through. Serve hot.

Apple and Pulled Pork Hash Cakes

Prep Time: 5 minutes

Cook Time: 10 minutes

Servings: 2

Hash cakes are a name of curious origin. The full name was hashed browned potatoes of which the first known mention was in the 1800's. Interestingly, the shortened name hash browns was used notably as early as 1959, by the main character in the pilot episode of The Twilight Zone. Do-do-do-do.....we call them hash cakes and ours with no spuds included are made into patties (or call them flying saucers if you like) of a delectable combination of apples and pulled pork.

INGREDIENTS

Hash Cakes:

8 oz pre-cooked pulled pork

1 tart apple

1 small white onion

1/4 – 1/2 cup almond flour

1 cage-free egg

Pinch ground black pepper

Pinch paprika

Pinch Celtic sea salt

Quick Grill Sauce:

8 oz (1 can) organic tomato sauce

1 sweet apple

2 whole roasted red peppers (jarred)

2 tablespoons organic mustard (or mustard powder)

1 tablespoon raw honey (optional)

1 oz apple cider vinegar

Pinch ground black pepper

Pinch paprika

Pinch cayenne pepper

Water

INSTRUCTIONS

1. Heat large skillet over medium-high heat and lightly coat with coconut oil. Heat small pot over medium heat.

2. Blend all **Quick Grill Sauce** ingredients in food processor or bullet blender. Only add as much water as needed to get mixture smooth. Add to small pot and reduce until thickened to BBQ sauce consistency.

3. Beat egg in medium bowl with black pepper, paprika and salt. Peel and core apple. Grate apple and onion and add to medium bowl.

4. Lightly shred pulled pork and add to bowl. Sprinkling in almond flour a little at a time and mix with hand or wooden spoon. Get pulled pork mixture to just hold together in patty form. Do not over-flour or over mix.

5. Form 2 large or 4 small patties and gently lay into hot oiled skillet. Cook about 2 - 3 minutes, until golden brown and crisp. Flip and cook another 2 - 3 minutes, or until heated through and browned.

6. Remove cooked patties from pan and drain on paper towel. Serve hot.

Ham, Egg & Veggie Breakfast Burrito

Prep Time: 10 minutes

Cook Time: 10 minutes

Servings: 2

You're going to enjoy this two-for-one recipe combo. Not only do you get the recipe for our filling ham, egg & veggie filling; you get the bonus of a great tortilla recipe too! Consider making a double batch of tortillas while you're at it for using with different fillings later. This filling is made with a combination of unbeatable ingredients when it comes to adding flavor and texture. We've included peppers and onions for crunch and salsa for that dance along flavor.

INGREDIENTS

Tortillas:

2 tablespoons coconut flour

2 tablespoons almond flour

2 teaspoons ground flax seed

2 eggs

2 tablespoons melted coconut oil

1/4 teaspoon baking powder

1/4 - 1/2 cup water

Coconut oil (for cooking)

Filling:

6 oz natural pre-cooked ham

6 cage-free eggs

1 bell pepper

1/2 red onion

1 avocado

4 oz organic salsa

Pinch Celtic sea salt

Pinch ground black pepper

INSTRUCTIONS

1. Heat large pan over medium-high heat and coat with 2 tablespoons of coconut oil. Heat second skillet over medium heat and lightly coat with coconut oil.

2. For *Tortillas*, blend coconut flour, almond flour, flax meal and baking powder in medium bowl. In separate bowl, whisk together 2 eggs, 2 tablespoons coconut oil and 1/4 cup water.

3. Slowly whisk dry blend into wet mixture. Whisk as you pour to avoid clumps. Continue to whisk and slowly add just enough water to make thin but hearty batter.

4. Once coconut oil is hot, use ladle or dry measure cup to pour half of batter into large pan. Tilt pan in circular motion as you pour so batter spreads thinly. Cook batter for about 2 minutes or until tortilla is slightly golden and firm.

5. While *Tortillas* cook, seed and stem pepper and peel onion. Chop ham, pepper and onion. Add to second skillet and sauté for about 2 minutes.

6. Flip tortilla and cook for 2 more minutes. Remove when toasted and cooked through. Place on paper towel or parchment. Add remaining batter to large pan, repeating tilting process to create thin tortilla.

7. While second tortilla cooks , beat 6 eggs in medium bowl and pour over veggies and ham. Salt and pepper to taste. Scramble until desired firmness.

8. Fill both tortillas down center each with half of ham scramble. Slice avocado in half, pit, then scoop out flesh onto each burrito.

9. Roll up tortillas and plate fold-side down. Dollop with your favorite salsa. Serve warm.

GF Breakfast Pizza

Prep Time: 10 minutes

Cook Time: 15 minutes

Servings: 2

Pizza for breakfast? YES. Pizza is always a kids favorite, but hey let's not "kid" ourselves; we love it too. We call this a breakfast pizza since it features sausage and eggs. It doesn't stop there though. Roasted red peppers give it pop and fresh herbs add a taste sensation that you can only get from the good earth itself. Enjoy this pizza equally as much for lunch or dinner too!

INGREDIENTS

Crust:

1 1/2 cup almond flour

1/4 cup tablespoons coconut flour

2 cage-free eggs

1 tablespoon melted coconut oil

Coconut oil (for cooking)

Topping:

4 eggs

4 oz pre-cooked natural sausage

1/2 small red onions

1 /2 green pepper

1 whole roasted red pepper (jarred)

Handful black olives

1 tablespoon rosemary

Pinch ground black pepper

Pinch Celtic sea salt

INSTRUCTIONS

1. Preheat oven to 425 degrees F. Heat medium skillet to medium heat and lightly coat with coconut oil. Coat 8 or 9-inch round cake pan with coconut oil and dust with coconut flour.

2. Combine all *Crust* ingredients in small bowl. If too soft, add 1 tablespoon of coconut flour at a time. If too firm, add 1 tablespoon of water at a time. Adjust until firm dough that can hold its shape forms.

3. Form dough into ball and place in cake pan. Gently pat it into 1/4 inch thick circle, building up around edge about 1/2 - 1 inch up sides of pan. Bake crust for 5 minutes.

4. Chop sausage and rosemary. Seed and stem green pepper and peel onion. Slice onion and pepper and add to skillet with sausage. Sauté about 2 minutes.

5. Whisk eggs in medium bowl and add eggs to skillet, plus rosemary. Remove skillet from heat and scramble very lightly.

6. Reduce oven to 350 degrees F and remove pan. Carefully pour runny scrambled eggs into crust. Slice roasted red pepper and olives and sprinkle over eggs. Salt and pepper to taste.

7. Return pizza to oven and bake another 10 - 15 minutes or until eggs firm.

8. Slice and serve hot from pan. Or remove, slice and serve.

Turkey Bacon Club Salad

Prep Time: 10 minutes

Cook Time: 5 minutes

Servings: 1

You're going to love having a "club" that you don't have to dislocate your jaw to bite into. I mean truly, haven't you ever wondered how a human being is supposed to take a bite of a club sandwich? There's no denying that this taste combination is popular for a good reason—it's delicious! Our version is every bit as delicious and even that much more satisfying with its gorgeous bed of romaine lettuce and a drizzle of luscious and creamy avocado dressing.

INGREDIENTS

Salad:

4 slices turkey bacon

1 tablespoon coconut oil

1 heart of romaine lettuce

2 medium tomatoes, chopped

Dressing:

1 avocado

1/2 small white onion

1 small garlic clove

Juice of 1 lemon

Small bunch of parsley leaves

Pinch Celtic sea salt

Pinch ground black pepper

INSTRUCTIONS

1. Heat medium skillet to medium-high heat and add coconut oil.

2. Chop turkey bacon and add to skillet. Browned for 2 - 3 minutes on each side, until thoroughly cooked. Remove turkey bacon and preserve any leftover oil.

3. Rinse and dry heart of romaine, then chop. Dice tomato and toss with lettuce in large bowl.

4. For **Dressing**, slice avocado in half, pit, and spoon flesh into food processor or bullet blender. Add peeled onion and garlic, lemon juice and parsley. Add excess coconut oil from pan. Process until smooth. Salt and pepper to taste.

5. Use tongs to transfer lettuce and tomatoes to plate. Sprinkle on turkey bacon, and drizzle with avocado **Dressing**. Serve immediately.

GF Cobb Salad

Prep Time: 10 minutes

Cook Time: 10 minutes

Servings: 1

Cobb salad is beautiful, with it's lively sections of brightly colored fresh ingredients all aligned like one big edible rainbow. Having the choice of which tidbits to combine in each mouthful makes it fun to eat as well. This healthy version uses only the best ingredients, cage-free eggs, natural ham and farm fresh produce to make it both nutritious and stunning to the eye. Try packing it for lunch and watch your coworkers eye you with envy!

INGREDIENTS

Salad:

2 slices natural ham

2 slices nitrate-free bacon

1 heart of romaine

1/2 cup watercress

1/2 cup spinach

1 medium tomato

1/2 avocado

1 cage-free egg

Dressing:

2 tablespoons coconut oil

1 tablespoon apple cider vinegar

1 tablespoon lime juice

1 teaspoon organic mustard (or powder)

1/2 avocado

1 small clove garlic,

Small bunch cilantro

Pinch Celtic sea salt

Pinch ground black pepper

Pinch paprika

Pinch cayenne pepper

INSTRUCTIONS

1. Bring small pot to boil with salted water. Heat medium skillet over medium-high heat.

2. Gently add whole egg to boiling water for about 7 minutes, or until hard boiled.

3. While egg cooks, chop bacon and ham. Add bacon pieces to skillet. Brown bacon for about 5 minutes, until crisp and cooked on both sides. Drain bacon on paper towel. Add ham to skillet just to warm, and remove skillet from heat. Stir to warm evenly.

4. Rinse and dry heart of romaine, spinach and watercress. Chop lettuce.

5. Dice tomato. Slice in half, pit and dice flesh of half of avocado. Reserve other half.

6. Drain warm ham on paper towel. Reserve leftover bacon grease.

7. Drain hardboiled egg and cool under running water for about 30 seconds. Peel egg and chop.

8. Peel onion and garlic. Then add all *Dressing* ingredients with reserved avocado half to food processor or bullet blender. Add

reserved bacon grease (optional). Process until smooth. Salt, pepper, paprika and cayenne to taste.

9. Use tongs to plate lettuce mix. Drizzle salad with avocado *Dressing*. Add chopped tomato, eggs, bacon, ham and avocado in single adjacent lines across lettuce mix. Serve immediately.

GF Crab Cakes

Prep Time: 5 minutes

Cook Time: 10 minutes

Servings: 2

The best crab cakes in town are now going to be found on your table! The trick is in keeping that beautiful lump crabmeat lumpy. By that, we mean make sure to leave lots of big succulent bites of crabmeat disbursed throughout the cake. A trick that you'll only find in the finest of restaurants. This is a dish that will become an all-time favorite and one of those dishes that's good enough to turn to for dinner meant to impress company.

INGREDIENTS

8 oz pre-cooked lump crabmeat

1 cage-free egg

1 lemon

1 teaspoon ground crab boil seasoning (Old Bay Seasoning™)

1 tablespoons fresh basil

1 tablespoon fresh parsley

1/4 cup almond meal

1 ripe avocado

Coconut oil (for cooking)

INSTRUCTIONS

1. Heat large skillet over medium-high heat and coat with coconut oil.

2. Slice in half, pit and scoop flesh of half of avocado into medium mixing bowl. Preserve other half.

3. Chop basil and parsley and add to avocado. Zest lemon into bowl to taste. Cut lemon in 1/2 and squeeze about 1 tablespoon of juice into bowl, excluding seeds. Mash well.

4. Add egg to bowl blend. Add crabmeat, crab boil seasoning and almond meal. Mix gently but thoroughly.

5. Form 4 small or 2 large crabmeat patties, pressing firmly to help hold them together. They will be delicate.

6. Add crab patties to hot oiled for about 3 - 4 minutes. Carefully flip and continue cooking for another 3 - 4 minutes on each side, or until golden brown.

7. Drain crab cakes on paper towel. Slice reserved avocado. Plate crab cakes and top with sliced avocado. Drizzle with squeeze of lemon. Serve hot.

No-Oats Oatmeal

Prep Time: 5 minutes

Cook Time: 10 minutes

Servings: 2

Huh, what is No-Oats Oatmeal? Sounds like all that's left is a bowl of mushy meal. You're in for a big surprise when you try this coconut milk based hot cereal chock full of fruit, nuts and seeds. It's really a bowl full of energy and a big hit with all who are lucky enough to sit down to it. What better way to get healthy carbs, fiber and protein all in one quick toothsome dish?

INGREDIENTS

2 cups coconut milk

1/2 cup quick tapioca

1/4 cup chia seed

1/2 cup dried dates

1 small banana

2 tablespoons slivered almonds

2 tablespoons pumpkin seeds

2 tablespoons flaked coconut

2 tablespoons walnuts

1 tablespoon vanilla

1 teaspoon ground cinnamon

2 tablespoons raw agave nectar (optional)

Pinch Celtic sea salt

Water

INSTRUCTIONS

1. Heat medium pan over medium heat .

2. Add almonds, pumpkin seeds, coconut flakes and walnuts to hot dry pan. Dry toast about 2 minutes, stirring frequently to prevent burning.

3. Pit and chop dates. Cut banana in half and blend with coconut milk and dates in food processor or bullet blender. Reserve other half of banana.

4. Add milk mixture to hot pan. Add quick tapioca, chia seeds, vanilla and pinch of salt. Stir and thicken over heat about 5 - 8 minutes, or until tapioca is soft. Add water to loosen for runnier "oatmeal."

5. Slice reserved half of banana. Serve hot in bowl. Top with banana slices, sprinkle with cinnamon, and drizzle with agave (optional).

Acorn Squash 'N Eggs

Prep Time: 5 minutes

Cook Time: 15 minutes

Servings: 2

Squirrel squash? No, of course not. This is farm fresh acorn squash that grows prolifically year-round and is full of flavor and nutrients. This is the perfect dish to play hide the veggie with if your little ones are inclined to boo hoo at the idea. Shredded and slightly caramelized, they resemble a small nest topped with a fresh egg. A simple and healthy way to put some gusto into anyone's step.

INGREDIENTS

1 medium acorn squash

2 cage-free eggs

1/2 small sweet onion

Ground black pepper, to taste

Celtic sea salt, to taste

1 tablespoon apple cider vinegar

Pinch of cinnamon (optional)

Coconut oil (for cooking)

INSTRUCTIONS

1. Heat large skillet over medium heat and coat generously with coconut oil. Bring medium pot to simmer with salted water, plus apple cider vinegar.

2. Peel acorn squash and onion, and grate. Drain shredding's in paper towel, pressing out moisture.

3. Combine squash, onion, black pepper and salt in small bowl. Place 4 handfuls into hot well-oiled skillet. Spread lightly to create thin, crisp patties. Brown acorn hash patties for about 5 minutes, then carefully flip. Brown another few minutes until cooked through.

4. While squash finishes, gently crack 1 egg into simmering water. Let poach for about 1 minute, then scoop out with slotted spoon and carefully drain on paper towel, careful to keep yolk intact. Repeat with second egg.

5. Plate acorn patties, 2 per person. Sprinkle with cinnamon (optional). Top with lightly poached egg. Remove from heat and serve.

Beef and Plantain Stir-Fry

Prep Time: 10 minutes

Cook Time: 15 minutes

Servings: 2

This dish says tortilla all over it! Of course that would be a GF tortilla (you can find the recipe in this book). Just as good served a la self on a nice warm plate, you'll enjoy spicy beef cubes along with onions, peppers and earthy seasonings. Tender plantains give a slightly sweet starchy bite and round out the party. Truly, it's like taking a trip south of the border inside your mouth.

INGREDIENTS

8 oz grass-fed beef

1 sweet plantain

1 small yellow onion

1/2 red bell pepper

2 cloves garlic

1 Serrano pepper

1 teaspoon ground cumin

1 teaspoon chili powder

1 teaspoon paprika

Small bunch fresh cilantro

1/2 lime

Coconut oil (for cooking)

INSTRUCTIONS

1. Bring a medium pot to boil with lightly salted water. Leave enough room in pot for sweet plantain. Heat large skillet over high medium heat and coat with coconut oil.

2. To peel plantain, cut in half then careful make at least 4 slices through peel lengthwise. Get finger or butter knife under tough peel and pry off.

3. Cut peeled plantain cut into 1 inch pieces, then in half, forming half moons. Add to boiling water for about 5 - 8 minutes, or until tender but not mushy.

4. Stem and seed peppers. Peel onion and garlic. Dice beef into half inch cubes and add to medium bowl. Mince Serrano pepper and garlic, and add to beef. Sprinkle with cumin, chili powder and paprika. Mix with wooden spoon to avoid getting hot pepper oil on skin.

5. Slice onion and bell pepper and add to hot skillet. Sauté about 1 minute. Add seasoned beef to skillet. Sauté another 2 minutes to brown.

6. Remove plantains from boiling water and drain. Add to hot skillet and stir-fry all together for about 2 - 3 minutes, until beef is browned and cook to about medium-well and plantains are a bit caramelized.

7. Chop fresh cilantro. Remove skillet from heat and toss stir-fry with cilantro. Plate stir-fry and squeeze over lime juice. Serve hot.

GF Tuna Spread

Prep Time: 5 minutes

Servings: 1

Spread it, stuff it, scoop it, dip it….just try not to wear it! You'll never get rid of the neighbor's cat. This delicious tuna mixture is so versatile that you can use it any way your imagination wanders. Kids adore this served in celery and men love it grilled as a patty served with a side of kale chips. Tuna is truly a wonder in a can. Make sure to keep this recipe hand for a quick party dip too!

INGREDIENTS

7oz (1 can) chunk light tuna

1 avocado

1/2 small red Onion

1 carrot

1 celery stalk

1/2 Lemon

1/2 cucumber

Ground black pepper, to taste

Celtic sea salt, to taste

Paprika, to taste

INSTRUCTIONS

1. Drain tuna. Cut celery stalk in half, and preserve larger end. Peel onion. Slice avocado in half, pit and scoop out flesh into small bowl. Mash well.

2. Finely dice onion, smaller half of celery stalk, and carrot. Add to bowl, with spices to taste.

3. Add tuna to bowl, plus squeeze of lemon. Mix until combined and smooth.

4. Slice reserved half of celery stalk into sticks. Slice cucumber into 1/3 inch round.

5. Serve tuna in bowl with cucumber chips and celery sticks.

GF Egg In A Hole

Prep Time: 5 minutes

Cook Time: 15 minutes

Servings: 2

First off, how in the world did the egg fall into a hole and how are you supposed to get it out-- tongs? All kidding aside, you'll find this recipe for GF Egg In A Hole to be yummy, quick and family-friendly. This is one of those fail-safe breakfast dishes that will prove to be a favorite of everybody. The best part is that GF Egg In A Hole is designed to fill you up with healthy goodness without any fuss or mess, plus it gives you a great presentation and a lot of mealtime fun too.

INGREDIENTS

Pancakes:

1 3/4 cups almond meal

3/4 cup almond milk

2 cage-free eggs

1 teaspoon baking powder

1 teaspoon vanilla

Pinch Celtic sea salt

Pinch ground black pepper

Agave nectar (optional)

Coconut oil (for cooking)

Filling:

4 cage-free eggs

INSTRUCTIONS

1. Heat large skillet with lid over medium heat and lightly coat with coconut oil.

2. Whisk together 2 eggs, almond milk and vanilla in medium bowl. Whisk in almond flour, baking powder and salt until smooth.

3. Use ladle or dry measure cup to pour 1/3 of batter onto hot oiled skillet in a circle with a hole large enough for one egg. Fit up to 2 pancakes comfortably, so they do not touch as they spread.

4. Crack one egg into each space within pancake. Cover with lid and cook until sides of pancakes are firm and batter bubbles up a bit. About 3 - 4 minutes.

5. Remove lid and gently flip pancakes with spatula, careful to keep yolks intact. Cook uncovered for about 3 minutes, or until pancakes are cooked through.

6. Repeat with remaining batter. Re-oil pan if necessary. Pancakes will be slightly delicate, so flip and plate with care.

7. Sprinkle egg with salt and pepper to taste. Drizzle with agave nectar (optional). Serve warm.

GF Apple Nut Bake

Prep Time: 5 minutes

Cook Time: 15 minutes

Servings: 2

If you've never heard of apple nuts, you're not alone. Truthfully that's just a silly play on words and this dish is delish. Apples and nuts are a naturally good combination and in this dish they bake together beautifully. First you'll poke through the nutty and crunchy cinnamon topping, and then work down into tender sweet and tart apples. This is a particularly good dish to make and take to get-togethers. Just don't plan on bringing home any leftovers.

INGREDIENTS

Filling:

2 sweet apples

2 tart apples

2 tablespoons almond flour

2 tablespoons flax meal

1 tablespoon sweetener*

1 tablespoons ground cinnamon

1 teaspoon ground nutmeg

1 teaspoon ground ginger

1 teaspoon vanilla

Pinch Celtic sea salt

Pinch ground black pepper

Topping:

2 tablespoons coconut oil

1/2 cup almonds

1/2 cup pecans

1/2 cup walnuts

1 tablespoon ground cinnamon

1 teaspoon ground nutmeg

1 tablespoon sweetener*

Pinch Celtic sea salt

Pinch ground black pepper

INSTRUCTIONS

1. Preheat oven to 400 degrees F and lightly oil square baking pan.
2. Peel, core and dice apples. Toss apples with all *Filling* ingredients in medium bowl. Pour into baking pan.
3. Process all *Topping* ingredients in food processor or bullet blender until crumbly. Sprinkle evenly over apples.
4. Bake 15 - 20 minutes, or until apples are soft and crust is crisp. Serve hot.

*stevia, raw honey, or agave nectar

Bacon & Fruit Scramble

Prep Time: 10 minutes

Cook Time: 15 minutes

Servings: 2

What an enticing way to celebrate figs, the fruit of Eden. Where there are leaves there must be fruit, don't you think? (It's best we leave the apple part of the discussion out of things here). These delicious morsels are featured along with apples, bacon and farm fresh eggs. Did you know that scrambling is the most popular way to prepare eggs? You'll find this to be an easy and quick way to celebrate the morning in a special way.

INGREDIENTS

6 cage-free eggs

4 slices nitrate-free bacon

2 dried figs

1 sweet apple

1 bell pepper

1 small sweet onion

1/2 teaspoon ground black pepper

1/2 teaspoon paprika

1/2 teaspoon Celtic sea salt

1/2 teaspoon cinnamon (optional)

INSTRUCTIONS

1. Bring small pot to boil with lightly salted water. Heat medium skillet over medium-high heat.

2. Dice bacon and add to hot skillet. Brown bacon for about 3 minutes, stirring occasionally with wooden spatula.

3. Add figs to boiling water for 5 minutes.

4. Peel and core apple. Stem and seed pepper. Peel onion. Dice apple, pepper and onion and add to skillet. Sauté another 2 minutes, until veggies caramelize and bacon crisps.

5. Remove figs from boiling water and dice. Add to skillet, plus spices. Sauté another minute.

6. Crack eggs directly into skillet and scramble gently with wooden spatula.

7. Cook eggs to desired firmness and serve hot.

Salmon & Veggie Breakfast Salad

Prep Time: 10 minutes

Cook Time: 10 minutes

Servings: 1

Oohs and aahs are all you'll hear when you set this beauty onto your table. Salmon is one of those ideal fish that gives you Omega 3's along with a stunning presentation. We've paired it up with a medley of crisp fresh vegetables featuring elegant asparagus. Serve it with our chilled avocado-herb dressing and you'll have a show stopper every time. As an added bonus, all of the salads elements can be prepared ahead of time and quickly assembled at meal time.

INGREDIENTS

Salad:

1 medium salmon fillet (or 2 oz smoked salmon, do not cook)

1 carrot

1/2 cucumber

8 asparagus stalks

1 cup cabbage

1/2 lemon

Dressing:

1 avocado

2 tablespoons coconut oil

1/2 lemon

1 small clove garlic

1 tablespoon fresh parsley

1 tablespoon fresh dill

Pinch Celtic sea salt

Pinch ground black pepper

Pinch paprika

INSTRUCTIONS

1. Bring small pot to boil with salted water. Heat small skillet over medium-high heat and lightly coat with coconut oil.

2. Parboil asparagus spears in boiling water for about 2 minutes. Then drain and shock in ice bath.

3. Lay salmon fillet skin-side down in hot oiled skillet. Cook about 3 minutes on each side. Season to taste, then squeeze lemon juice over fillet.

4. Shred or grate cabbage, carrot and cucumber. Drain cucumber in paper towel. Dry asparagus in paper towel and slice into 2 inch pieces. Toss veggies together.

5. Peel garlic and add all *Dressing* ingredients with squeeze of lemon and salt, pepper and paprika to taste to food processor or bullet blender. Process until smooth.

6. Plate shredded veggies. Remove salmon fillet and flake off meat over shredded veggies. Or lay smoked salmon slices over veggies.

7. Drizzle salad with avocado *Dressing*. Squeeze a little more lemon juice over salad. Serve immediately.

Kids Lunch Recipes

Pita Bites

Prep Time: *5 minutes

Cook Time: 20 minutes

Servings: 1

Kids love foods they can dip, and hummus is a favorite with kids near and far. With its mild taste and smooth texture it pleases many palates. These little bread bites are perfect for scooping up just the right amount of this creamy dip.

INGREDIENTS

Pita Bites

1 cup tapioca flour/starch

1 teaspoon ground chia seed (or flax meal)

1 egg

2 tablespoons vegetable oil

1/4 cup water

1/2 teaspoon baking soda

1/4 teaspoon salt

Almond Hummus

1 cup skinless almonds

1/3 cup tahini

1 garlic clove

Juice of 1/2 lemon

Zest of 1/2 lemon

1/4 teaspoon salt

1/4 cup water

2 tablespoons pine nuts

INSTRUCTIONS

1. *Soak almonds overnight in enough water to cover. Drain and rinse.

2. Preheat oven to 375 degrees F. Cover sheet pan with parchment paper or baking mat. Heat small pot over low heat.

3. For *Pita Bites*, mix 1/3 cup tapioca flour with chia meal, water and 1 tablespoon coconut oil in pot. Stir until mixture comes together. Remove from heat and cool in freezer.

4. In medium bowl, blend remaining tapioca flour, baking soda and salt. Then add egg and remaining oil. Mix until combined.

5. Add cooled chia mixture to bowl and mix to combine. Then remove and knead to form dough.

6. Form large round disk, then use rolling pin to flatten on lined baking sheet. Cut out circles with biscuit cutter or drinking glass, or cut triangles with pizza cutter. Re-roll excess dough and repeat until all dough is used.

7. Arrange pita pieces on sheet pan and place in oven. Bake about 10 minutes. Carefully turn over with spatula and bake another 5 - 7 minutes, or until crisp.

8. Remove from oven and let cool completely. Place in lidded container or sealable lunch bag and serve room temperature.

9. For *Almond Hummus*, add 1/2 of water to all ingredients in food processor or bullet blender and process. Add just enough water to smooth blend.

10. Scrape hummus into lidded container and serve chilled or room temperature with *Pita Bites*.

Homemade Applesauce

Prep Time: 10 minutes

Cook Time: 20 minutes

Servings: 4

Show kids that applesauce doesn't grow in jars. Incredibly easy to make, even kids can help in the process. The result is so full of the flavor of apples and sweet spices you will never go back to the packaged variety.

INGREDIENTS

2 sweet apples

2 tart apples

1/4 cup sweetener*

3/4 cup water

1/2 teaspoon ground cinnamon

1/4 teaspoon ground ginger

INSTRUCTIONS

1. Peel, core and chop apples. Add to medium pan with sweetener, water and spices. Stir to combine.
2. Cover pan with lid, and heat pan over medium heat. Cook apples about 20 minutes. Transfer to heat-safe bowl and let cool about 5 minutes.
3. Mash apples with fork or potato masher. Then chill in refrigerator.
4. Transfer chilled applesauce to lidded container. Serve chilled or room temperature.

Banana Pudding

Prep Time: 5 minutes

Cook Time: 15 minutes

Servings: 4

This is a favorite of southern cuisine. Replace the artificially flavored boxed stuff with this homemade versions to really appreciate how good this old-fashioned delight can be.

INGREDIENTS

3 overripe bananas

13 oz (1 can) full-fat coconut milk

2 egg yolks

1 tablespoon coconut oil

1 tablespoon almond butter (or cashew butter)

1 teaspoon vanilla

1 teaspoon ground cinnamon

INSTRUCTIONS

1. Heat medium pan over medium heat. Heat small pot over medium heat.
2. Add coconut milk, egg yolks and vanilla to pot and whisk until mixture starts to thicken. Remove from heat.
3. Add coconut oil and nut butter to pan. Add bananas and cinnamon, mashing a bit. Allow bananas to cook and caramelize slightly.
4. Pour thickened coconut milk mixture into food processor or blender. Add banana mixture and process until smooth.

5. Pour creamy pudding into serving bowls or lidded containers. To prevent skin from forming, lay sheet of plastic wrap directly over surface of serving bowls. Or secure lids on containers.

6. Refrigerate about 1 hour. Serve chilled.

Pizza Bites

Prep Time: 20 minutes*

Cook Time: 20 minutes

Servings: 4

Mini pizza pies are a perennial favorite and are a feature at many kids'
parties. These tasty bites are as fun and delicious as the frozen ones.
Topped with quality meats, this is a high-protein lunch that kids will love.

INSTRUCTIONS

Crust

2 cups almond flour

2 eggs

3 tablespoons vegetable oil

1/4 teaspoon baking soda

1 teaspoon salt

Almond Cheese

1 cup skinless almonds*

1/4 cup water

2 tablespoons vegetable oil

1 tablespoon lemon juice

1 tablespoon apple cider vinegar

1 garlic clove

1/2 teaspoon salt

1/4 teaspoon ground white pepper (or black pepper)

Pizza Sauce

4 oz tomato paste

4 oz GF tomato sauce

1 teaspoon dried oregano

1/2 teaspoon dried basil

1/2 teaspoon ground black pepper

Filling

4 oz GF pepperoni

4 oz GF ground sausage

1/2 bell pepper

DIRECTIONS

1. *For *Almond Cheese*, soak almonds in 1 1/2 cups water overnight. Drain and rinse.

2. For *Crust*, sift almond flour into medium mixing bowl. Add baking soda, spices and salt.

3. Whisk eggs in small mixing bowl, then add to flour and combine. Slowly add coconut oil until malleable dough comes together.

4. Roll in plastic wrap or wrap tightly in parchment and refrigerate for 15 minutes.

5. Preheat oven to 400 degrees. Line sheet pan with parchment or baking mat. Cover cutting board with parchment. Heat medium pan over medium heat.

6. Seed and stem bell pepper. Dice pepper and pepperoni. Add peppers and sausage to hot pan. Sauté about 5 minutes, until sausage is cooked through. Transfer to small bowl to cool, and add diced pepperoni. Set aside.

7. Add all *Almond Cheese* ingredients to food processor or bullet blender and process until smooth. Add a few extra tablespoons of water if necessary to achieve thick but smooth consistency. Set aside.

8. In small bowl, mix together all *Pizza Sauce* ingredients. Set aside.

9. Remove dough from refrigerator. Roll dough out on parchment covered cutting board with rolling pin to about 1/8 inch thickness. Use sharp knife or pizza cutter to cut dough into 2x4 inch rectangles.

10. Spread *Almond Cheese* in center of one half of each dough piece. Then dollop with small amount of *Pizza Sauce*, and a pinch of *Filling*.

11. Fold over bare half of dough. Press edges together, pressing out any trapped air. Use fork to crimp edges for better seal. Repeat with remaining dough.

12. Arrange *Pizza Bites* on lined sheet pan and bake 15 - 20 minutes, or until dough is golden and cooked through.

13. Serve immediately. Or allow to cool and store in air-tight container.

Soft Baked Pretzel

Prep Time: 15 minutes

Cook Time: 20 minutes

Servings: 4

Chewy, salty, and satisfying--pretzels are a delicious snack or side dish.
Try dipping them in a mild mustard for an old-world style treat.

INGREDIENTS

1 cup coconut flour

1/2 cup tapioca flour/starch

1/2 cup vegetable oil

1/2 cup water

1 egg

2 tablespoon apple cider vinegar

1/2 teaspoon baking soda

1/2 teaspoon baking powder

1/2 teaspoon salt

INSTRUCTIONS

1. Preheat oven to 350 degrees F. Heat medium pan over medium-high heat. Line sheet pan with parchment or baking mat.

2. Add coconut oil, water, vinegar and salt to pot. Bring to a boil and remove from heat.

3. Whisk in tapioca flour. Stir with wooden spoon or soft spatula until mixture gels and comes together.

4. Stir in baking soda and baking powder. Continue mixing for a minute. Mixture will foam and expand. Let mixture sit and cool about 5 minutes.

5. Sift in coconut flour. Mix partially, then beat in egg. Blend until combined. Excess coconut flour may sit in bottom of bowl.

6. Turn out dough onto cutting board dusted with any excess coconut flour from mixture. Knead dough for 2 minutes.

7. Cut dough into 4 equal portions. Roll out pieces into ropes and twist to form classic pretzel twist. Pinch together any crumbled dough.

8. Arrange pretzels on lined sheet pan. Brush with coconut oil or full-fat coconut milk and sprinkle with salt.

9. Place sheet pan in oven and bake about 25 minutes, until cooked through.

10. Serve immediately with organic mustard. Or allow to cool and serve room temperature.

Frontier Anzac Biscuits

Prep Time: 5 minutes

Cook Time: 25 minutes

Servings: 4

Anzac biscuits are a favorite sweet cookie in Australia and New Zealand—originally created to send in care packages to troops in the First World War. Traditional Anzac biscuits are made without eggs, due to wartime shortages, but they do contain oats, which are off-limits on most GF diets. With the crunchy almonds and coconut flakes here you won't miss them!

INGREDIENTS

3/4 cup almond flour

3/4 cup sliced almonds

3/4 cup coconut flakes

1/4 cup sweetener*

1/4 cup coconut oil

1/2 teaspoon baking soda

1 tablespoon water

INSTRUCTIONS

1. Preheat oven to 300 degrees F. Line sheet pan with parchment sheet or baking mat.
2. In medium mixing bowl, combine almond flour, sliced almonds and coconut flakes.

3. Mix baking soda and water in small mixing bowl. Add to medium mixing bowl with sweetener and oil. Mix until combined. Add water 1 tablespoon at a time if dough is too crumbly.

4. Form 12 large biscuits and arrange on sheet pan. Flatten slightly with hand for even baking.

5. Bake for 25 - 30 minutes, until golden.

6. Serve immediately. Or allow to cool completely and pack in airtight container or sealable baggie.

* raw honey or agave nectar

Cream Filled Carrot Cake Muffin

Prep Time: 10 minutes*

Cook Time: 20 minutes

Servings: 12

Cream-filled cakes are one of the delights of childhood. In this modern version the mild flavor of carrots is enhanced by cinnamon and mellowed with the yummy cream filling.

INGREDIENTS

1 1/2 cups almond flour

2 tablespoons tapioca flour

2 eggs

 4 - 6 carrots (1 1/2 cups grated)

1/4 cup coconut oil

1/2 cup unsweetened applesauce

1/4 cup sweetener*

1 teaspoon baking soda

1 teaspoon baking powder

1 tablespoon ground cinnamon

1 teaspoon vanilla

1/2 teaspoon salt

Cashew Cream Filling

1 cup cashews

2 - 4 tablespoons sweetener**

1 teaspoon cinnamon

1 1/2 cups water

INSTRUCTIONS

1. *Soak cashews in 1 1/2 cups water overnight. Drain and rinse.

2. Preheat oven to 350 degrees F. Line muffin pan with paper liners or coconut oil.

3. Grate or chop carrot in food processor or bullet blender until coarsely ground. Add to medium mixing bowl with eggs, oil, applesauce and sweetener and beat with hand mixer or whisk.

4. Sift in almond flour, baking soda, baking powder, spices and salt. Mix to combine.

5. Use ice cream scoop or tablespoon to scoop batter into muffin tins 1/2 - 2/3 full.

6. Bake 15 - 18 minutes until muffins are golden brown and tops are firm to the touch.

7. Remove muffins from oven and let cool about 10 minutes.

8. For *Cashew Cream*, process soaked cashews, sweetener and cinnamon in food processor or bullet blender. Add water 1 tablespoon at a time if necessary, just to smooth.

9. Cut hole in top of muffin about 1 inch deep and spoon in *Cashew Cream*. Or fill pastry bag fitted with 1/2 inch tip with Cashew Cream, and inject muffin with cream.

10. Serve warm or room temperature.

**stevia, raw honey or agave nectar*

Sausage Stuffed "Corn" Muffin

Prep Time: 10 minutes

Cook Time: 20 minutes

Servings: 12

Here's a savory snack that is a huge improvement on "corn dogs," but preserves that salty, smoky flavor. These are great at snack time—also perfect for picnics and lunchboxes. They even make a tasty breakfast! Get your little cowpokes filled up and ready to go!

INGREDIENTS

1 cup almond flour

2 eggs

1/4 cup coconut oil

2 tablespoons unsweetened applesauce

1 teaspoon sweetener*

1 teaspoon apple cider vinegar

1 teaspoon baking powder

1/2 teaspoon ground turmeric

1/2 teaspoon ground white pepper (optional)

Filling

8 oz GF ground sausage (or GF sausage patties)

2 teaspoons ground sage

INSTRUCTIONS

1. Preheat oven to 350 degrees F. Line muffin pan with paper liners or lightly coat with coconut oil. Heat small skillet over medium-high heat.

2. Add sausage and sage to skillet and sauté about 5 - 8 minutes, until cooked through. Break up sausage if in patties.

3. Beat eggs in medium mixing bowl with hand mixer or whisk until thick and slightly foamy. Add oil, applesauce, sweetener and vinegar. Mix well.

4. Stir in almond meal, baking powder, turmeric and pepper until combined.

5. Use ice cream scoop or tablespoon to scoop batter into muffin tins, about 1/4 - 1/3 full. Spoon sausage over batter. Then top with second scoop of batter. Fill each muffin cup only 1/2 - 2/3 full.

6. Bake 15 - 18 minutes until edges are golden brown and tops are firm.

7. Serve warm. Or allow to cool and serve room temperature.

stevia, raw honey or agave nectar

Baby BLT

Prep Time: 15 minutes

Cook Time: 25 minutes

Servings: 4

Introduce your kids to the classics early on! And what could be more classic than this simple sandwich—made more fun here and easier to eat for smaller hands. The bacon-y dressing puts a new spin on it for the younger generation.

INGREDIENTS

Sandwich Bread

1 cup tapioca flour/starch

1/4 - 1/3 cup coconut flour

1 egg

1/2 cup warm water

1/4 cup vegetable oil

1/4 cup applesauce

1 teaspoon apple cider vinegar

1/2 teaspoon baking soda

1/2 teaspoon salt

Bacon Dressing

Bacon drippings

1/4 cup vegetable oil

2 tablespoons mustard

Filling

8 strips nitrate-free bacon

1 tomato

4 romaine lettuce leaves

INSTRUCTIONS

1. Preheat oven to 350 degrees F. Line sheet pan with parchment paper or coat with vegetable oil.

2. In medium bowl, sift together tapioca flour, 1/4 cup coconut flour, baking soda and salt. Stir in warm water and oil.

3. Whisk egg in small bowl. Add applesauce and vinegar. Then add egg mixture to flour mixture and mix until well combined. Add 1 tablespoon coconut flour or water at a time if needed to form soft and slightly sticky dough.

4. Divide dough into 4 portions and roll into round or oval balls. Dust your hand with extra tapioca flour to prevent sticking.

5. Place rolls on sheet pan and pat down slightly. Bake 20 - 25minutes, or until edges are golden brown and the tops are firm. Remove from oven and allow to cool.

6. While *Sandwich Bread* is baking, heat large skillet over medium-high heat. Cut bacon strips in half and add to hot pan. Cook bacon until crisp and cooked through. Set aside.

7. For *Bacon Dressing*, add excess bacon grease to food processor or bullet blender with coconut oil and mustard. Blend until light and emulsified.

8. Slice tomatoes. Rinse and dry lettuce, then chop. Slice cooled *Sandwich Bread* in half and spread on *Bacon Dressing*. Layer a few slices of bacon, tomatoes and lettuce pieces on bread.

9. Serve immediately. Or wrap in plastic wrap or parchment and store in lidded container.

Cheese Steak Sandwich

Prep Time: 15 minutes*

Cook Time: 25 minutes

Servings: 4

Philadelphia claims the honor of having invented the cheese steak sandwich. The meaty, cheesy specialty inspires hot debates among fans over just who makes the best one in the city. You will hold the title in your town when you serve this version to the little ones!

INGREDIENTS

Sandwich Bread

1 cup tapioca flour/starch

1/4 - 1/3 cup coconut flour

1 egg

1/2 cup warm water

1/4 cup vegetable oil

1/4 cup applesauce

1 teaspoon apple cider vinegar

1/2 teaspoon baking soda

1 teaspoon salt

Almond Cheese

1 cup skinless almonds*

2 tablespoons coconut oil (or walnut oil)

1 tablespoons lemon juice

1 tablespoon apple cider vinegar

1 garlic clove

1/4 teaspoon ground white pepper (or black pepper)

1/2 teaspoon salt

1/4 cup water

Filling

8 oz beef steak

1 small onion

1/2 bell pepper

1/2 teaspoon ground black pepper

1/2 teaspoon salt

INSTRUCTIONS

1. *Soak almonds in enough water to cover overnight. Drain and rinse.
2. Preheat oven to 350 degrees F. Line sheet pan with parchment paper or coat with vegetable oil.
3. In medium bowl, sift together tapioca flour, 1/4 cup coconut flour, baking soda and salt. Stir in warm water and oil.
4. Whisk egg in small bowl. Add applesauce and vinegar. Add egg mixture to flour mixture and mix until well combined. Add 1 tablespoon coconut flour or water at a time if needed to form soft and slightly sticky dough.
5. Divide dough into 3 portions and roll into loaves. Dust your hand with extra tapioca flour to prevent sticking.

6. Place loaves on sheet pan and pat down slightly. Bake 20 - 25minutes, or until edges are golden brown and the tops are firm. Remove from oven and allow to cool.

7. While *Sandwich Bread* is baking, add all *Almond Cheese* ingredients to food processor or bullet blender and process until smooth. Add 1 tablespoon of water at a time to reach preferred consistency.

8. Heat medium skillet over medium-high heat. Add 1 tablespoon coconut oil to hot pan.

9. Thinly slice steak, onion and pepper. Add steak to hot pan and sauté about 1 minute. Add veggies, salt and pepper. Sauté about 5 minutes, until meat is cooked and veggies are soft and caramelized. Remove from heat and set aside.

10. Slice cooled *Sandwich Bread* in half and spread on *Almond Cheese*. Layer meat and veggies on bread.

11. Serve immediately. Or wrap in plastic wrap or parchment and store in lidded container.

Cashew Butter and Banana Sandwich

Prep Time: 10 minutes

Cook Time: 20 minutes

Servings: 4

This is so good that you will want to pack one for yourself! Cashews and bananas are really wonderful together, and the hint of cinnamon in the sandwich bread pulls it all together. Smooth, sweet, and silky textured, these could easily become a favorite.

INGREDIENTS

Sandwich Bread

1 cup tapioca flour/starch

1/4 - 1/3 cup coconut flour

1 egg

1/2 cup warm water

1/4 cup vegetable oil

1/4 cup applesauce

1 tablespoon sweetener*

1 teaspoon apple cider vinegar

1/2 teaspoon baking soda

1/2 teaspoon cinnamon

1/2 teaspoon salt

Filling

1/2 cup cashews (raw or roasted)

2 tablespoons oil

1 tablespoon sweetener*

1/4 teaspoon cinnamon

1 banana

INSTRUCTIONS

1. Preheat oven to 350 degrees F. Line sheet pan with parchment paper or coat with coconut oil.

2. In medium bowl, sift together tapioca flour, 1/4 cup coconut flour, baking soda and salt. Stir in warm water and oil.

3. Whisk egg in small bowl. Add applesauce, vinegar and cinnamon. Add egg mixture to flour mixture and mix until well combined. Add 1 tablespoon coconut flour or water at a time if needed to form soft and slightly sticky dough.

4. Divide dough into 4 portions and roll into round or oval balls. Dust your hand with extra tapioca flour to prevent sticking.

5. Place rolls on sheet pan and pat down slightly. Bake 20 minutes, or until edges are golden brown and the tops are firm. Remove from oven and allow to cool.

6. While *Sandwich Bread* is baking, add cashews, coconut oil, sweetener and cinnamon to food processor or bullet blender and process until smooth. Add 1/2 tablespoon of coconut oil at a time if necessary to reach preferred consistency. Or use jarred cashew butter.

7. Slice bananas. Slice cooled *Sandwich Bread* in half and spread on cashew butter. Layer banana slices on bread.

8. Serve immediately. Or wrap in plastic wrap or parchment and store in lidded container.

*stevia, raw honey or agave nectar

Almond Butter and Strawberry Sandwich

Prep Time: 10 minutes

Cook Time: 20 minutes

Servings: 4

A slightly more sophisticated take on the standard PB&J. This one uses the good stuff: rich almond butter, fresh strawberries, and a touch of ginger. It gives this familiar taste combo an exotic flair. It is lovely to look at too!

INGREDIENTS

Sandwich Bread

1 cup tapioca flour/starch

1/4 - 1/3 cup coconut flour

1 egg

1/2 cup warm water

1/4 cup vegetable oil

1/4 cup applesauce

1 tablespoon sweetener*

1 teaspoon apple cider vinegar

1/2 teaspoon cinnamon

1/4 teaspoon ground ginger

1/2 teaspoon baking soda

1/2 teaspoon salt

Filling

1/2 cup almonds (raw or roasted)

2 tablespoons coconut oil

1 tablespoon sweetener*

1/4 teaspoon cinnamon

1/4 teaspoon ground ginger

5 - 6 medium strawberries

INSTRUCTIONS

1. Preheat oven to 350 degrees F. Line sheet pan with parchment paper or coat with coconut oil.

2. In medium bowl, sift together tapioca flour, 1/4 cup coconut flour, baking soda and salt. Stir in warm water and oil.

3. Whisk egg in small bowl. Add applesauce, vinegar, cinnamon and ginger. Add egg mixture to flour mixture and mix until well combined. Add 1 tablespoon coconut flour or water at a time if needed to form soft and slightly sticky dough.

4. Divide dough into 4 portions and roll into round or oval balls. Dust your hand with extra tapioca flour to prevent sticking.

5. Place rolls on sheet pan and pat down slightly. Bake 20 minutes, or until edges are golden brown and the tops are firm. Remove from oven and allow to cool.

6. While *Sandwich Bread* is baking, add almonds, coconut oil, sweetener, cinnamon and ginger to food processor or bullet blender and process until smooth. Add 1/2 tablespoon of coconut oil at a time if necessary to reach preferred consistency. Or use jarred almond butter.

7. Slice strawberries. Slice cooled *Sandwich Bread* in half and spread on almond butter. Layer strawberry slices on bread.

8. Serve immediately. Or wrap in plastic wrap or parchment and store in lidded container.

*stevia, raw honey or agave nectar

Beef Bun

Prep Time: 15 minutes

Cook Time: 30 minutes

Servings: 4

Slightly spicy—these beefy patties put a little fiesta in lunchtime. They are a bit like the Cornish pasties of British cuisine, but here they take on some south-of-the-border seasonings for a zesty change. Excellent alternative when you want to enliven things a little.

INGREDIENTS

Bun

1 cup tapioca flour/starch

1/4 - 1/3 cup coconut flour

1 egg

1/2 cup warm water

1/2 cup coconut oil

1 teaspoon apple cider vinegar

1/2 teaspoon baking soda

1 teaspoon salt

Filling

8 oz ground beef

1/2 small onion

1 garlic clove

1 teaspoon ground cumin

1/2 teaspoon chili powder

1/4 teaspoon cayenne

1/2 teaspoon ground black pepper

1/2 teaspoon salt

INSTRUCTIONS

1. Preheat oven to 350 degrees F. Line sheet pan with parchment paper or coat with coconut oil. Heat medium skillet over medium-high heat.

2. For *Filling*, grind or mince onion and add to skillet with beef, salt and spices. Sauté until cooked through and browned, about 8 - 10 minutes. Remove from heat and set aside.

3. In medium bowl, sift together tapioca flour, 1/4 cup coconut flour, baking soda and salt. Stir in warm water and oil.

4. Whisk egg and vinegar in small bowl. Add egg mixture to flour mixture and mix until well combined. Add 1 tablespoon coconut flour or water at a time if needed to form soft and slightly sticky dough.

5. Divide dough into 4 portions and flatten into round disks. Dust your hand or rolling pin with extra tapioca flour to prevent sticking.

6. Scoop beef filling into center of dough disks and pinch edged of dough together to create round, sealed ball.

7. Place buns sealed side down on sheet pan and pat down slightly. Bake 20 minutes, or until edges are golden brown and dough is cooked through.

8. Serve immediately. Or store in lidded container.

Cocoa Cream Bun

Prep Time: 10 minutes

Cook Time: 20 minutes

Servings: 4

The rich chocolate cake and the vanilla cream center in this special treat will spread good cheer. Like the ones you had when you were a kid—without the wrapper! Or all the junk. Everyone will be smiling.

INGREDIENTS

Bun

1 cup tapioca flour/starch

1/4 - 1/3 cup coconut flour

1 egg

1/2 cup warm water

1/2 cup vegetable oil

1 tablespoon sweetener*

1 teaspoon apple cider vinegar

1 tablespoon cocoa powder

1/2 teaspoon cinnamon

1/2 teaspoon baking soda

1/2 teaspoon salt

Filling

1 cup cashews (raw or roasted)

2 tablespoons coconut cream

2 tablespoons coconut oil

2 tablespoons cocoa powder

3 tablespoons sweetener*

1/2 teaspoon cinnamon

INSTRUCTIONS

1. Preheat oven to 350 degrees F. Line sheet pan with parchment paper or coat with coconut oil. Heat medium skillet over medium-high heat.

2. For *Filling*, add cashews, coconut oil, coconut cream, cocoa powder, sweetener and cinnamon to food processor or bullet blender and process until smooth. Add 1/2 tablespoon coconut oil at a time if needed to reach desired consistency. Set aside.

3. In medium bowl, sift together tapioca flour, 1/4 cup coconut flour, cocoa powder, cinnamon, baking soda and salt. Stir in warm water and oil.

4. Whisk egg in small mixing bowl. Add sweetener and vinegar. Add egg mixture to flour mixture and mix until well combined. Add 1 tablespoon coconut flour or water at a time if needed to form soft and slightly sticky dough.

5. Divide dough into 4 portions and flatten into round disks. Dust your hand or rolling pin with extra tapioca flour to prevent sticking.

6. Scoop *Filling* into center of dough disks and pinch edges of dough together to create round, sealed ball.

7. Place buns sealed side down on sheet pan and pat down slightly. Bake 20 minutes, or until edges are golden brown and dough is cooked through.

8. Serve immediately. Or store in lidded container.

*stevia, raw honey or agave nectar

Honey Nut Bun

Prep Time: 15 minutes

Cook Time: 30 minutes

Servings: 4

Grocery aisles are filled with cereals and pastries that combine the taste of nuts and honey. They just naturally go together. Serve these sticky sweet buns as an after lunch treat, and they will be busy as bees all afternoon.

INGREDIENTS

Bun

1 cup tapioca flour/starch

1/4 - 1/3 cup coconut flour

1 water

1/2 cup coconut oil

1 teaspoon apple cider vinegar

1 teaspoon vanilla

1/2 teaspoon cinnamon

1/2 teaspoon baking soda

1/2 teaspoon salt

Filling

1 cup walnuts

1/4 cup sweetener*

2 teaspoons cinnamon

1 teaspoon ground ginger

INSTRUCTIONS

1. Preheat oven to 350 degrees F. Line sheet pan with parchment paper or coat with coconut oil. Heat medium skillet over medium-high heat.

2. For *Filling*, mix walnuts, sweetener, cinnamon and ginger in small mixing bowl. Set aside.

3. In medium bowl, sift together tapioca flour, 1/4 cup coconut flour, vanilla, cinnamon, baking soda and salt. Stir in warm water and oil.

4. Whisk egg and vinegar in small bowl. Add egg mixture to flour mixture and mix until well combined.

5. Add 1 tablespoon coconut flour or water at a time if needed to form soft and slightly sticky dough.

6. Divide dough into 4 portions and flatten into round disks. Dust your hand or rolling pin with extra tapioca flour to prevent sticking.

7. Scoop *Filling* into center of dough disks and pinch edges of dough together to create round, sealed ball.

8. Place buns sealed side down on sheet pan and pat down slightly. Bake 20 minutes, or until edges are golden brown and dough is cooked through.

9. Serve immediately. Or store in lidded container.

*stevia, raw honey or agave nectar

Chicken Pot Pie

Prep Time: 15 minutes

Cook Time: 30 minutes

Servings: 4

Chicken pot pie is just home-style yumminess served in a bowl. The addition of dried thyme to the pastry takes it beyond the ordinary. This pie is hearty and satisfying and on a cold day nothing could be better than this.

INGREDIENTS

Filling

8 oz skin-on chicken

1 1/2 cup GF chicken broth

2 tablespoons tapioca flour

2 tablespoons vegetable oil

2 carrots

1 celery stalk

1 green bell pepper

1 small onion

2 garlic cloves

2 teaspoons dried thyme (or 4 teaspoons fresh thyme)

1 tablespoon lemon juice

1/2 teaspoon black pepper

Pinch salt

Crust

1/3 cup almond flour

2 tablespoons coconut flour

3 tablespoons cold coconut oil (or cacao butter)

1 egg

3 - 4 teaspoons water

1/2 teaspoon dried thyme

1/4 teaspoon salt

INSTRUCTIONS

1. Preheat oven to 400 degrees F. Heat medium pot over medium heat.

2. Add two tablespoon coconut oil to hot pot. Add chicken pieces skin side down. Cook about 3 minutes, then turn with tongs and continue cooking another 3 minutes. Remove chicken and set aside.

3. Whisk coconut flour into pot until smooth. Gradually whisk in chicken broth. Simmer about 5 minutes, whisking occasionally.

4. Peel and mince garlic. Chop carrots, celery, onion and bell pepper. Add to pot with thyme, salt pepper and lemon juice.

5. Chop par-cooked chicken meat. Add back to pot and simmer for 5 minutes. Remove from heat and set aside.

6. For *Crust*, add cold coconut oil to flours, thyme and salt in small bowl. Cut fat into flour with fork until crumbly. Mix in egg and enough water to bring together tender dough.

7. Divide dough into 4 portions. Roll into balls and flatten into round disks large enough to fit over mini pie tins or ceramic ramekins with hand, then rolling pin.

8. Pour *Filling* into vessels and cover with crusts. Pinch edges of dough over edges of vessels to seal in liquid. Brush top of each pie with coconut oil, coconut milk, or egg wash and sprinkle with salt. Use knife to cut a slit in the top of each pie.

9. Bake pot pies for about 15 minutes, until crust is golden.

10. Remove from oven and allow pies to cool for 10 minutes.

11. Serve warm. Or let cool completely and serve room temperature.

Lamb Pot Pie

Prep Time: 15 minutes

Cook Time: 30 minutes

Servings: 4

Expand some culinary horizons with this tasty dish. With its sweet peppers and flavorful spices, it will remind you of middle eastern cuisines. Introduce your kids to the wonders of world cuisines with this mellow and satisfying meal.

INGREDIENTS

Filling

8 oz lamb

1 1/2 cup beef or vegetable broth

2 tablespoons tapioca flour

2 tablespoons coconut oil

2 chopped carrots

1 chopped celery stalk

1 bell pepper (yellow, orange or red)

1 small green tomato (or under ripe red tomato)

1 small onion

2 garlic cloves

1 inch piece ginger

1 tablespoon curry powder

1 tablespoon ground coriander

1 teaspoon ground cumin

1/2 teaspoon ground cinnamon

1/2 teaspoon black pepper

Pinch Celtic sea salt

Crust

1/3 cup almond flour

2 tablespoons coconut flour

3 tablespoons cold coconut oil (or cacao butter)

1 cage-free egg

3 - 4 teaspoons water

1/2 teaspoon turmeric

1/4 teaspoon salt

INSTRUCTIONS

1. Preheat oven to 400 degrees F. Heat medium pot over medium heat.
2. Add two tablespoon coconut oil to hot pot. Add lamb. Sauté about 5 minutes, then remove lamb with tongs.
3. Whisk in coconut flour until smooth. Gradually whisk in broth. Simmer about 5 minutes, whisking occasionally.
4. Peel and mince garlic and ginger. Chop carrots, celery, onion, bell pepper and tomato. Add to pot with salt, and spices.
5. Chop par-cooked lamb meat. Add lamb back to pot and simmer for 5 minutes. Remove from heat and set aside.
6. For *Crust*, add cold coconut oil to flours, turmeric and salt in small bowl. Cut fat into flour with fork until crumbly. Mix in egg and enough water to bring together tender dough.

7. Divide dough into 4 portions. Roll into balls and flatten into round disks large enough to fit over mini pie tins or ceramic ramekins with hand, then rolling pin.

8. Pour *Filling* into vessels and cover with crusts. Pinch edges of dough over edges of vessels to seal in liquid. Brush top of each pie with coconut oil, coconut milk, or egg wash and sprinkle with salt. Use knife to cut a slit in the top of each pie.

9. Bake pot pies for about 15 minutes, until crust is golden.

10. Remove from oven and allow pies to cool for 10 minutes.

11. Serve warm. Or let cool completely and serve room temperature.

My Favorite Meatballs

Prep Time: 5 minutes

Cook Time: 20 minutes

Servings: 4

These meatballs will quickly become favorites in your home too! These make a great meal with a vegetable side dish, or can be served as a snack. For extra fun, try serving them with picks—just don't let them roll out the door!

INGREDIENTS

16 oz (1 lb) ground meat (beef, pork, chicken, bison, or any combination)

1 cup almond flour

1 egg

1 garlic clove

1/2 small onion

1 teaspoon dried parsley

1 teaspoon dried oregano

1/2 teaspoon ground black pepper

1/2 teaspoon salt

Tomato Sauce

4 oz GF tomato sauce

4 oz crushed tomatoes

1 teaspoon dried oregano

1/2 teaspoon dried basil

1/2 teaspoon ground black pepper

DIRECTIONS

1. Preheat oven to 350 degrees. Line baking sheet with parchment or baking mat. Or prepare glass or ceramic casserole dish.

2. Pulse onion and garlic in food processor or blender until finely processed, but before paste forms. Or finely mince onion and garlic.

3. Beat egg in large bowl. Add ground meat, almond flour, spices and salt. Mix well with hands or large wooden spoon.

4. Form 18 - 24 meatballs with scoop or tablespoon, then roll in hands.

5. Arrange meatballs on lines sheet pan or in casserole dish and bake for 15 to 20 minutes, until golden brown and cooked through.

6. Add all *Tomato Sauce* ingredients to small pot and heat over medium heat. Stir and simmer about 10 minutes, until reduced and thickened.

7. Remove meatballs from oven. Toss with *Tomato Sauce* and serve hot.

8. Or allow meatballs and *Tomato Sauce* to cool, then pack in lidded containers. Serve room temperature.

Bacon Baked Apples

Prep Time: 15 minutes

Cook Time: 30 minutes

Servings: 4

These lush apples would be perfect at a holiday lunch with their dried fruit centers and sweet and smoky juices. Don't save them just for autumn days!

INGREDIENTS

6 oz nitrate-free bacon (thick slices or whole slab)

4 tart apples

4 dried apricots

2 tablespoons dried cranberries

2 tablespoons dried cherries

2 tablespoons dried raisins

1 tablespoon cinnamon

Juice of half a lemon

Zest of half a lemon

Water

INSTRUCTIONS

1. Preheat oven to 350 degrees F. Heat medium skillet over medium-high heat.
2. Chop apricots. Add dried fruit to small bowl with lemon juice. Add enough water just to cover fruit. Let fruit rehydrate for 10 minutes.

3. Dice bacon and add to hot skillet. Sauté about 5 - 8 minutes, until crisp and golden brown.

4. Slice apples in half lengthwise. Carefully core apples, scooping out seeds, stem and tough core with melon baller. Leave good-sized well in apple.

5. Arrange apples in baking dish just large enough to fit them snuggly. Pour water into bottom of baking dish, about 1/8 inch.

6. Strain fruit, reserving liquid in small bowl. Strain bacon, reserving liquid. Mix lemon zest, cinnamon and bacon with fruit.

7. Fill apple wells with fruit mixture. Press down into apple, packing slightly.

8. Pour 1 teaspoon reserved liquid and over each apple. Follow by 1 tablespoon bacon grease over all 8 apple halves.

9. Bake in preheated oven for 20 - 30 minutes, until apples are tender.

10. Serve warm. Or allow to cooled completely, and store in lidded container.

Peach Pecan "Fried" Pie

Prep Time: 20 minutes

Cook Time: 20 minutes

Servings: 4

Peachy keen and sweet as pie—what a combination! Peaches and pecans—traditional southern crops--come together in these hand held pies— and they just taste like summer. Find a shady spot and a cool drink and savor the moment.

INSTRUCTIONS

Crust

2 cups almond flour

2 eggs

3 tablespoons coconut oil

1 tablespoon sweetener*

1/4 teaspoon baking soda

1 teaspoon ground cinnamon

1/2 teaspoon salt

Filling

2 peaches

1/4 cup dried apricots

1/4 cup pecans

2 tablespoons sweetener*

2 tablespoons water

1 tablespoon ground cinnamon

1 teaspoon vanilla

1/2 teaspoon ground ginger

DIRECTIONS

1. Preheat oven to 400 degrees. Line sheet pan with parchment or baking mat. Cover cutting board with parchment.

2. For *Crust*, sift almond flour into medium mixing bowl. Add baking soda, cinnamon and salt.

3. Whisk eggs and sweetener in small mixing bowl, then add to flour and combine. Slowly add coconut oil until malleable dough comes together.

4. Roll in plastic wrap or wrap tightly in parchment and refrigerate for 15 minutes.

5. Heat medium pan over medium heat.

6. Peel and pit peaches. Chop apricots, pecans and peaches. Add to hot pan with sweetener, spices and water. Sauté about 5 - 10 minutes, until peaches are tender and

7. Remove dough from refrigerator. Roll dough out on parchment covered cutting board to about 1/8 inch thick square with rolling pin. Use sharp knife or pizza cutter to cut dough into 4 squares.

8. Scoop equal portions of *Filling* into center of one side of each dough square. Fold bare half of dough over filled half. Press edges together, letting any trapped air escape. Crimp edges of dough together with fork. Repeat with remaining dough.

9. Arrange pies on lined sheet pan and bake 15 - 20 minutes, or until dough is golden and cooked through.

10. Serve immediately. Or allow to cool and store in air-tight container.

stevia, raw honey or agave nectar

NOTE: Heat large skillet over medium heat , add 1/4 inch coconut oil, and fry pies 2 minutes on each side for traditional *Fried Pies*.

Sweet Potato "Fried" Pie

Prep Time: 20 minutes

Cook Time: 30 minutes

Servings: 4

Sweet potato pie is often served at Thanksgiving along with the pumpkin and mince, but there's no reason to restrict these little gems to the holiday table. Kids will love the bright orange color and the crispy fried crust.

INSTRUCTIONS

Crust

2 cups almond flour

2 eggs

3 tablespoons coconut oil

1 tablespoon sweetener*

1/4 teaspoon baking soda

1/2 teaspoon ground cinnamon

1/2 teaspoon salt

Filling

1 large sweet potato

1/2 cup dried dates

1/4 cup walnuts

1 egg

1 teaspoon vanilla

1 teaspoon ground cinnamon

1 teaspoon ground nutmeg

1/2 teaspoon ground black pepper

DIRECTIONS

1. Bring medium pot of lightly salted water to boil. Cover cutting board with parchment.

2. For *Crust*, sift almond flour into medium mixing bowl. Add baking soda, cinnamon and salt.

3. Whisk eggs and sweetener in small mixing bowl, then add to flour and combine. Slowly add coconut oil until malleable dough comes together.

4. Roll in plastic wrap or wrap tightly in parchment and refrigerate for 15 minutes.

5. Preheat oven to 400 degrees. Line sheet pan with parchment or baking mat.

6. Peel and dice sweet potato. Chop dates. Add sweet potato and dates to boiling water peaches. Cook about 10 minutes, until sweet potatoes are soft. Drain sweet potatoes and dates.

7. Add egg to medium mixing bowl. Add 1 tablespoon hot sweet potatoes to bowl. Mash briefly, then add second tablespoon. Gradually add all hot sweet potatoes and dates to egg. Mash and mix, careful not to scramble egg. Stir in vanilla, cinnamon, nutmeg and pepper.

8. Chop walnuts. Set aside.

9. Remove dough from refrigerator. Roll dough out on parchment covered cutting board to about 1/8 inch thick square with rolling pin. Use sharp knife or pizza cutter to cut dough into 4 squares.

10. Scoop equal portions of *Filling* into center of one side of each dough square. Fold bare half of dough over filled half. Press edges

together, letting any trapped air escape. Crimp edges of dough together with fork. Repeat with remaining dough.

11. Arrange pies on lined sheet pan and bake 15 - 20 minutes, or until dough is golden and cooked through.

12. Serve immediately. Or allow to cool and store in air-tight container.

stevia, raw honey or agave nectar

NOTE: Heat large skillet over medium heat , add 1/4 inch coconut oil, and fry pies 2 minutes on each side for traditional *Fried Pies*.

Asian Empanada

Prep Time: 20 minutes

Cook Time: 20 minutes

Servings: 4

Fusion food at its best! This east-meets-west pastry will draw universal raves. Sort of like an egg roll, but with the tender crust of the Latin favorite, the combination works beautifully. Best eaten with your hands!

INSTRUCTIONS

Crust

1 cup almond flour

1 cup coconut flour

2 eggs

3 tablespoons sesame oil (or coconut oil)

1/2 teaspoon garlic powder

1/2 teaspoon onion powder

1/2 teaspoon ground ginger

1/4 teaspoon baking soda

1 teaspoon salt

1 tablespoon sesame oil (or coconut oil)

1 tablespoon sesame seeds

Filling

6 oz chicken or shrimp

1/2 head cabbage (1 cup shredded)

1 carrot

1/4 cup mushrooms

2 inch piece fresh ginger

2 garlic cloves

1 tablespoon pure GF fish sauce

1 teaspoon apple cider vinegar

1 shallot

1 scallion

1 teaspoon sesame oil

DIRECTIONS

1. For *Crust*, sift almond and coconut flour into medium mixing bowl. Add baking soda, spices and salt.

2. Whisk eggs in small mixing bowl, then add to flour and combine. Slowly add 3 tablespoons oil until malleable dough comes together.

3. Roll in plastic wrap or wrap tightly in parchment and refrigerate for 15 minutes.

4. Preheat oven to 400 degrees. Line sheet pan with parchment or baking mat. Cover cutting board with parchment. Het medium pan over medium heat.

5. Shred cabbage, grate carrot, slice mushrooms. Peel and grate ginger. Slice scallion. Peel and mince shallot and garlic. Dice chicken or slice shrimp in half.

6. Add sesame oil to pan. Add chicken or shrimp hot oiled pan with ginger, shallot and garlic. Sauté about 90 seconds. Add cabbage, carrot, and mushrooms and sauté for a minute.

7. Add vinegar and fish sauce. Sauté about 3 minutes until cabbage is wilted. Stir in scallions. Remove from heat and set aside.

8. Remove dough from refrigerator. Divide dough into 4 portions. Roll dough into balls and flatten on parchment covered cutting board with hands. Roll into circles about 1/8 inch thick with rolling pin.

9. Scoop equal portions of *Filling* into center of one side of dough circle. Fold bare half of dough over filled half. Press edges together, letting any trapped air escape. Crimp edges of dough together with fork. Repeat with remaining dough.

10. Bruch tops of empanada with sesame oil and sprinkle with sesame seeds.

11. Arrange empanadas on lined sheet pan and bake 15 - 20 minutes, or until dough is golden and cooked through.

12. Serve immediately. Or allow to cool and store in air-tight container.

Jamaican Jerk Patty

Prep Time: 20 minutes

Cook Time: 30 minutes

Servings: 4

Jerk is a Caribbean style of cooking that uses spices to create a unique flavor blend. It always includes hot pepper, allspice, and cinnamon—as does the meat filling in these pies. If you haven't used allspice before, it is a sweet spice similar to nutmeg. You can find it ground in the spice section of any grocery store. This hot meat filling is mellowed by the rich pastry crust in a perfect combination. Serve with fruit salad for a taste of the Islands!

INSTRUCTIONS

Crust

2 cups almond flour

2 eggs

3 tablespoons coconut oil

1 teaspoon GF curry powder

1/4 teaspoon baking soda

1/2 teaspoon salt

Filling

8 oz meat (ground or shredded chicken, beef or pork)

1 small onion

1 tablespoon GF curry powder

1 teaspoon allspice

1 teaspoon chile powder

1 teaspoon cayenne pepper

1 teaspoon red pepper flake

1/2 teaspoon garlic powder

1/2 teaspoon onion powder

1/2 teaspoon ground cinnamon

DIRECTIONS

1. For *Crust*, sift almond flour into medium mixing bowl. Add baking soda, curry powder and salt.

2. Whisk eggs in small mixing bowl, then add to flour and combine. Slowly add coconut oil until malleable dough comes together.

3. Roll in plastic wrap or wrap tightly in parchment and refrigerate for 15 minutes.

4. Preheat oven to 400 degrees. Line sheet pan with parchment or baking mat. Cover cutting board with parchment. Heat medium pan over medium heat.

5. Peel and mince onion. Add to hot pan with ground or shredded meat and spices. Sauté about 5 - 10 minutes, until beef is browned. Remove from heat and set aside.

6. Remove dough from refrigerator. Divide dough into 4 portions. Roll dough into balls and flatten on parchment covered cutting board with hands. Roll into circles about 1/8 inch thick with rolling pin.

7. Scoop equal portions of *Filling* into center of one side of dough circle. Fold bare half of dough over filled half. Press edges together, letting any trapped air escape. Crimp edges of dough together with fork. Repeat with remaining dough.

8. Arrange patties on lined sheet pan and bake 15 - 20 minutes, or until dough is golden and cooked through.
9. Serve immediately. Or allow to cool and store in air-tight container.

Chicken Tenders

Prep Time: 5 minutes

Cook Time: 10 minutes

Servings: 2

What kid doesn't love chicken tenders? They will love these too—and so will you. No fillers, no mystery meats, no questionable additives. Just pure, finger-licking good chicken—perfect with the not-too-sweet honey mustard dip.

INGREDIENTS

8 oz boneless, skinless chicken

1 egg

1/2 cup almond meal

1 teaspoon flax meal

1 teaspoon paprika

1/2 teaspoon thyme

1/2 teaspoon onion powder

1/2 teaspoon ground black pepper

1/2 teaspoon salt

Vegetable oil for frying

Honey Mustard

2 tablespoon raw honey or agave nectar

3 tablespoons mustard

INSTRUCTIONS

1. Heat a medium skillet over medium high heat. Lightly coat pan with vegetable oil.

2. Slice chicken into 1 inch wide strips. Arrange slices between 2 sheets of parchment and pound with kitchen mallet or rolling pin to flatten slightly. Place flattened pieces between two paper towels to absorb excess moisture.

3. In a shallow dish, blend almond meal, flax meal, spices and salt.

4. Beat egg in small mixing bowl. Dip chicken into beaten egg, then dredge in seasoned almond meal.

5. Carefully place coated chicken strips into hot oil and fry about 3 - 4minutes, until golden brown and cooked through. Turn with tongs half way through cooking.

6. Drain cooked chicken on paper towel, then transfer to serving dish. Serve warm.

7. Or allow to cool and transfer to lidded container. Serve room temperature or chilled.

8. Mix mustard and sweetener in small serving bowl or lidded container. Serve with chicken for dipping.

stevia, raw honey or agave nectar

Turkey Tenders

Prep Time: 5 minutes

Cook Time: 15 minutes

Servings: 2

These will be "gobbled" up in no time! Turkey makes a nice change from chicken, without being too challenging to picky eaters. The cranberry compote makes this a fun feast any time of the year.

INGREDIENTS

8 oz boneless skinless turkey

1 egg

1/2 cup almond meal

1 teaspoon flax meal

1/4 teaspoon garlic powder

1/2 teaspoon paprika

1/2 teaspoon ground sage

1/2 teaspoon ground black pepper

1/2 teaspoon salt

Vegetable oil for frying

Cranberry Compote

1/4 cup dried cranberries

1 teaspoon sweetener*

1/2 teaspoon arrowroot powder (or tapioca flour)

1/2 cup water

INSTRUCTIONS

1. Heat a medium skillet over medium high heat. Lightly coat pan with vegetable oil. Heat small pot over medium heat. Add 1/2 cup water and bring to boil.

2. Slice turkey into 1 inch wide strips. Arrange slices between 2 sheets of parchment and pound with kitchen mallet or rolling pin to flatten slightly. Place turkey between two paper towels to absorb excess moisture.

3. Blend almond meal, flax meal, spices and salt in a shallow dish.

4. Beat egg in small mixing bowl. Dip turkey strips into beaten egg, then dredge in seasoned almond meal.

5. Carefully place coated turkey into hot oil and fry about 3 - 4 minutes, until golden brown and cooked through. Turn half way through cooking with tongs.

6. Add cranberries to boiling water, and whisk in sweetener and arrowroot or tapioca. Reduce heat to medium and stir occasionally as compote thickens, about 5 - 8 minutes.

7. Drain cooked turkey on paper towel, then transfer to serving dish. Serve warm.

8. Or allow to cool and transfer to lidded container. Serve room temperature or chilled.

9. Pour *Cranberry Compote* into small serving bowl or lidded container. Serve with chicken.

*stevia, raw honey or agave nectar

Snack Recipes

Spicy Chicken Bites

Trust me, these go down easy! Totally addicting—spicy, savory, crunchy—they hit all the right spots! Make lots and freeze for a perfect quick bite any time hunger strikes.

Prep Time: 5 minutes

Cook Time: 10 minutes

Servings: 4

INGREDIENTS

8 oz boneless skinless chicken

1/2 cup almond meal

1 teaspoon flax meal

1 teaspoon paprika

1/2 teaspoon cayenne pepper

1/2 teaspoon red pepper flakes

1/2 teaspoon ground black pepper

1/2 teaspoon salt

1 egg

1 jalapeño pepper

2 garlic cloves

2 oz GF spicy brown mustard

Vegetable oil (for cooking)

INSTRUCTIONS

1. Heat a medium skillet over medium high heat. Lightly coat pan with oil.

2. Slice chicken into 1x1 inch strips. Arrange slices between 2 sheets of parchment and pound with kitchen mallet or rolling pin to flatten slightly. Place flattened pieces between two paper towels to absorb excess moisture.

3. In a shallow dish, blend almond meal, flax meal, dry spices and salt.

4. Add egg, jalapeño and peeled garlic to food processor or bullet blender. Process until fairly smooth. Pour into shallow dish.

5. Dip chicken pieces into jalapeño egg, then dredge in seasoned almond meal.

6. Carefully place coated chicken pieces into hot oil and fry about 2 minutes, until golden brown and cooked through. Turn with tongs half way through.

7. Drain cooked chicken on paper towel, then transfer to serving dish.

8. Serve hot with spicy mustard.

Highland Scotch Egg

Once upon a time, these little powerhouses were objects of ridicule. They seemed to represent everything that was heavy and stuffy about British cooking. Boy, do times change! Now we know that not only are these outrageously yummy, but they are incredibly portable and packed with protein to take the edge off hunger and fatigue.

Prep Time: 10 minutes

Cook Time: 25 minutes

Servings: 6

INGREDIENTS

6 eggs

12 oz GF ground sausage (pork, chicken, etc.)

1 tablespoon dried parsley

2 teaspoons lemon zest

1/4 teaspoon ground nutmeg

1/4 teaspoon dried sage

Pinch sea

Pinch ground black pepper

1 egg

1/2 cup almond meal

Vegetable oil (for cooking)

Mustard Sauce

1 egg yolk

1/4 cup vegetable oil

1/4 cup GF mustard

2 tablespoons sweetener*

INSTRUCTIONS

1. Bring medium pot of lightly salted water to boil.
2. Carefully place eggs in pot with tongs. Boil eggs for about 10 minutes.
3. For *Mustard Sauce*, add yolk, vegetable oil, mustard, and sweetener to food processor and bullet blender. Process until emulsified, about 2 minutes. Transfer to serving dish and refrigerate about 15 minutes.
4. Heat small pot over medium heat. Add enough vegetable oil to cover width of whole egg, about 2 1/2 inches.
5. Drain eggs and cool under cold running water. Once cool, peel off shells and set aside.
6. Add sausage to medium bowl with parsley, lemon zest, nutmeg, sage, salt and pepper. Mix to combine.
7. Wet hands and cover each whole, peeled egg with a layer of seasoned sausage. Work sausage around eggs and pat into even layer.
8. Pour almond meal into shallow dish. Whisk egg in small bowl. Roll sausage covered eggs in beaten egg, then dredge in almond meal.
9. Carefully place 2 eggs into hot oil and fry for 4 to 5 minutes, until browned and heated through. Turn half way through cooking with tongs.

10. Remove eggs with tongs or slotted spoon and place on paper towel to drain. Repeat with remaining eggs.
11. Serve hot with *Mustard Sauce*.

stevia, raw honey or agave nectar

NOTE: For *Baked Scotch Eggs*, preheat oven to 400 degrees F and bake coated eggs on wire rack over sheet pan for about 15 minutes, until sausage is fully cooked.

Jalapeño Bacon Bites

These flavorful bites will remind you of those cheesy jalapeño poppers everyone loves to gobble up at games and tailgate parties. If cheese and breading are off-limits now, you can still enjoy the bite of the hot pepper and the creaminess of melting cheesiness in this totally GF alternative.

Prep Time: 15 minutes
Cook Time: 20 minutes
Servings: 4

INGREDIENTS
6 medium to large jalapeño peppers
6 strips GF bacon
12 - 24 wooden toothpicks

Nut Cream Cheese
1/2 cup skinless almonds
1/2 cup cashews
2 tablespoons vegetable oil
1 tablespoon lemon juice
1 tablespoon apple cider vinegar
1 garlic clove
1/4 teaspoon ground white pepper (or black pepper)
1/2 teaspoon salt

INSTRUCTIONS

1. Soak toothpicks in water for about 5 minutes.

2. Peel garlic, and add all *Nut Cream Cheese* ingredients to food processor or bullet blender. Process until smooth. If necessary, let mixture sit for a few minutes, then continue to process to reach desired consistency.

3. Preheat oven to 375 degrees F. Place oven-safe wire rack over sheet pan.

4. Slice jalapeños in half lengthwise. Remove stems, seeds and veins. Cut bacon strips in half.

5. Fill jalapeño wells with *Nut Cream Cheese*, then wrap in half slice of bacon. Use 1 or 2 toothpicks per jalapeño to secure bacon.

6. Place bacon wrapped pepper on wire rack filling side up and place in oven. Bake for about 15 - 20 minutes, or until bacon is crisp. Remove and let cool about 2 minutes.

7. Serve warm or room temperature.

Fried Green Tomatoes

Maybe you remember this line from the book, *Fried Green Tomatoes at the Whistle Stop Cafe*--"I wonder how many people don't get the one they want, but end up with the one they're supposed to be with." Living GF is a little bit like that. Celebrate with the one you're *supposed* to be with by cooking up a batch of these southern fried favorites and enjoying life's little twists of fate. You won't miss the others!

Prep Time: 5 minutes

Cook Time: 15 minutes

Servings: 4

INGREDIENTS

2 large green tomatoes

Pinch salt

Pinch ground black pepper

Vegetable oil (for cooking)

Coating

1 cup almond flour

1 tablespoon tapioca flour

1 tablespoon ground chia seed (or flax meal)

1 egg

1/2 cup nutmilk

1/4 cup almond meal

1/4 cup almonds

1/4 teaspoon ground black pepper

1/2 teaspoon salt

INSTRUCTIONS

1. Heat medium pan over medium heat. Add 1/2 inch worth of vegetable oil.
2. Slice tomatoes into 1/2 inch thick slices. Discard ends.
3. Grind 1/4 cup almonds into course meal in food processor or bullet blender. Do not process into almond butter. Add to 1/4 cup almond meal, 1/4 teaspoon black pepper and 1/2 teaspoon salt in shallow dish.
4. In separate dish, combine almond flour, tapioca flour, and chia or flax meal.
5. Whisk eggs and milk together in small mixing bowl.
6. Dip tomato slices into flour mixture to coat. Then into the egg and milk mixture. Then dredge into almond meal mixture.
7. Carefully place 4 or 5 well coated tomatoes at a time into hot oil. Fry tomatoes for 2 -3 minutes on each side, until golden. Drain on paper towel and repeat with remaining tomatoes.
8. Serve hot.

Bacon Mofongo

Mofongo is a much-loved favorite in the Caribbean Isles. Its exact place of origin may be a matter of heated dispute among its many *aficionados*, but a few things are agreed on. Green plaintains are a must, and so are crispy, crackly, pork bits—and here bacon is put to perfect use. This is great any time of day, but is especially adored after a night of dancing and reveling.

Prep Time: 15 minutes

Cook Time: 15 minutes

Servings: 2

INGREDIENTS

1 green plantain

2 slices GF bacon

3 garlic cloves

1/4 teaspoon ground black pepper

Bacon drippings

Vegetable oil (for cooking)

INSTRUCTIONS

1. Bring medium pot of lightly salted water to boil.
2. Cut plantains into 1 inch slices. Remove peel and add to boiling water. Boil plantains for about 10 minutes, until soft.

3. Heat small pot over medium heat. Dice bacon and add to pot. Sauté and render out fat for about 5 minutes, until bacon is crisp. Pour bacon and drippings into medium bowl to cool slightly.

4. Add 1 inch worth of vegetable oil to hot pot.

5. Add slightly cooled bacon and drippings to food processor or bullet blender with peeled garlic. Process until well blended. Add back to medium bowl. Drain plantains and add to bowl with black pepper.

6. Mash plantains and seasonings in bowl with fork or potato masher. Roll mixture into 6 small balls.

7. Carefully add plantain balls to hot oil and fry for about 2 minutes. Turn with tongs half way through cooking. Remove and drain on paper towel.

8. Serve hot.

NOTE: For *Baked Mofongo*, preheat oven to 400 degrees F and bake plantain balls on oiled or parchment covered sheet pan for about 10 minutes, until golden brown.

Guilt-Free Guacamole

Guacamole is a favorite for so many reasons, not least of which that it's always been gluten-free—no need to change a thing to enjoy it! With the GF tortilla recipe here, or other GF chips or crackers, guacamole is always a safe and popular option when you're looking for a versatile item for picnics, cocktail parties, or potlucks. This is a classic variation that everyone will love.

Prep Time: 5 minutes
Cook Time: 5 minutes
Servings: 4

INGREDIENTS

2 avocados

1 shallot

1 small tomato

1 bunch cilantro

Half lime

2 teaspoons paprika

1/2 teaspoon ground cumin

1/2 teaspoon ground black pepper

1/2 teaspoon salt

INSTRUCTIONS

1. Peel and finely dice shallot. Dice tomato and cilantro. Add to small mixing bowl.

2. Slice avocados in half, pit, and scoop flesh into bowl. Add 1 teaspoon paprika, 1/2 teaspoon cumin, 1/2 teaspoon black pepper and 1/2 teaspoon salt.

3. Mash avocado and mix ingredients well with fork. Transfer to serving dish and squeeze on juice of half a lime. Sprinkle with remaining teaspoon of paprika.

4. Serve immediately. Or refrigerate 30 minutes, and serve chilled. Serve with GF tortillas or crackers or vegetable crudités.

Coconut Shrimp

Everyone loves coconut shrimp! What could be better? Crunchy, coconut, delights! These really go the extra mile in the coconut department—with coconut oil used to pan-fry the shrimp, and a thick crispy coating, coconut is more than just a suggestion here!

Prep Time: 10 minutes

Cook Time: 15 minutes

Servings: 4

INGREDIENTS

3 egg whites

1 lb large shrimp

1 cup flaked coconut

1/2 teaspoon garlic powder

1/2 teaspoon ground white pepper (or ground black pepper)

1 teaspoon salt

Vegetable oil, preferably coconut oil (for cooking)

Mango Salsa

1 ripe mango

1/2 small white onion

1 small jalapeño

Juice of half lime

INSTRUCTIONS

1. Preheat oven to 425 degrees F. Line sheet pan with parchment paper. Or place oven-safe wire rack over sheet pan.
2. Add coconut to shallow dish.
3. Beat egg whites with salt, pepper and garlic powder in a large mixing bowl with hand mixer or whisk until light and fluffy.
4. Peel and devein shrimp. Leave tails on. Add shrimp to egg whites to coat.
5. Let excess egg white drain from shrimp, then place in coconut flakes. Toss to coat. Return shrimp to egg whites, then coconut flakes again. Press shrimp into coconut and coat well.
6. Place the shrimp on prepared sheet pan. Brush lightly with liquid coconut oil.
7. Place in oven and bake for 5 - 7 minutes. Then turn shrimp over, brush with coconut oil, and bake another 5 - 7 minutes, until coconut is golden brown and shrimp are bright pink.
8. For *Mango Salsa*, slice mango around pit. Peel and dice flesh. Peel and dice onion. Mince jalapeño, discarding seeds and stem. Add to small serving dish juice of half a lime. Mix to combine.
9. Remove shrimp from oven and allow to cool for a few minutes.
10. Serve warm with *Mango Salsa*.

Green Deviled Eggs 'N Ham

Maybe you can't eat these quirky Dr. Seuss-inspired stuff eggs in a tree or on a boat, but enjoy these hearty egg-meat-and-veggie surprises for breakfast, lunch, or an afternoon snack, and you *will* indeed eat green deviled eggs n' ham!

Prep Time: 5 minutes

Cook Time: 10 minutes

Servings: 4

INGREDIENTS

8 eggs

1 avocado

1/2 teaspoon ground black pepper

1/2 teaspoon salt

2 oz GF ham

2 tablespoons fresh dill

INSTRUCTIONS

1. Bring medium pot of lightly salted water to boil. Gently add eggs to hot water with tongs and cook about 8 - 10 minutes.
2. Drain eggs in colander and cool in cold water.
3. Crack shells and peel eggs. Cut eggs in half lengthwise and scoop out yolks into small bowl. Arrange whites on platter with center hollows facing up.

4. Mash avocado, salt and pepper with egg yolks until smooth. Dice ham and dill, separately.

5. Scoop avocado blend into each egg white hollow and sprinkle with ham, then dill.

Refrigerate about 20 minutes. Serve chilled.

Piggies in a Poke

With a swanky cocktail, this groovy 1970s favorite never missed a party!
Invite them back into the swing of things by replacing that doughy old
blanket with a cool new wrap and really get the party started.

Prep Time: 20 minutes

Cook Time: 15 minutes

Servings: 4

INGREDIENTS

1 package(26 count) GF mini frankfurters

3 egg whites

1/4 cup almond flour

1/4 cup coconut flour

1 tablespoon cold coconut oil

1/2 teaspoon baking powder

Pinch garlic powder

Pinch salt

2 oz GF mustard

INSTRUCTIONS

1. In separate medium bowl, mix almond and coconut flours with
   baking powder. Cut-in cold coconut oil, then add pinch of
   garlic powder and salt. Mixture should be crumbly.
   Refrigerate 15 - 20 minutes.

2. Preheat oven to 400 degrees F. Line sheet pan with parchment or lightly coat with vegetable oil.

3. Whisk egg whites in medium bowl until white and frothy, just before soft peaks develop.

4. Gently fold egg whites into refrigerated flour mixture until just combined.

5. Flatten 1 level teaspoon of dough into a rectangle in your fingers. Place one frankfurter in middle of dough wrap it around the frankfurter. Repeat with remaining frankfurters and dough.

6. Place wrapped frankfurters on prepared sheet pan and bake about 15 minutes, until dough is golden brown and links are heated through.

7. Serve hot with mustard.

Mighty Beef Sliders

Mighty and mini might seem like a contradiction in terms—but like "jumbo shrimp" these tiny temptations pack a lot of taste in a small package. Filled with a spicy meaty center, these are just the thing for a big appetite!

Prep Time: 15 minutes

Cook Time: 25 minutes

Servings: 4

INGREDIENTS

Mini Burger Buns

1 1/2 cup raw cashews

1/3 cup coconut flour

1/4 cup almond flour

3 egg yolks

3 egg whites

1/4 cup vegetable oil

1/4 cup nutmilk

1 teaspoon apple cider vinegar

1 teaspoon baking soda

1 teaspoon salt

Filling

8 oz ground meat (beef, chicken, turkey, etc.)

1 teaspoon ground black pepper

1 teaspoon paprika

1/2 teaspoon salt

1/2 small onion

1 mini dill pickle (or 1/2 large dill pickle)

GF mustard

INSTRUCTIONS

1. Preheat oven to 325 degrees F. Line sheet pan with parchment paper or coat with vegetable oil.

2. Preheat oven.

3. Place cashews, egg yolks, nutmilk, vegetable oil and vinegar in a food processor or bullet blender. Process until smooth. Add coconut flour, almond flour and salt. Process again until a smooth, wet dough forms.

4. Beat egg whites in medium bowl with hand mixer until stiff peaks form. Add wet dough to egg whites with and blend until combined.

5. Wet hands and shape dough into 12 mini buns, similar to burger patties. Wet hands in between each bun.

6. Place buns on prepared sheet pan and bake for 10 -15 minutes, until golden and cooked through.

7. Heat large skillet or griddle over medium-high heat.

8. Mix ground meat with spices. Form into 12 mini patties. Place burgers on hot skillet or griddle and cook about 5 minutes, or until medium-well. Flip half way through cooking.

9. Remove buns from oven and allow to cool about 5 minutes.

10. Slices bun in half. Thinly slice onion and pickle. Place hamburger on bottom half of bun. Top with onion and pickle. Add mustard to taste. Top with top bun.

11. Serve warm.

Zucchini Rollatini

This is a real treat. These elegant fresh zucchini rolls are stuffed with oozing, melting, herby goodness! These are great as a satisfying snack or make a terrific light meal with some sliced meats and a salad. *Buon apetito*!

Prep Time: 15 minutes*
Cook Time: 25 minutes
Servings: 4

INGREDIENTS
Zucchini Pasta
1 large zucchini
Pinch salt
Pinch ground black pepper

Cashew Ricotta
1 cup cashews
1 1/2 cups water
2 teaspoons fresh basil
1 teaspoon ground white pepper (or black pepper)
1/2 teaspoon garlic powder
1/2 teaspoon salt

Pasta Sauce
6 oz (1 can) tomato paste

1/4 cup water

1 garlic clove

1 tablespoon oregano

2 teaspoons paprika

1 teaspoon ground black pepper

1/2 teaspoon salt

INSTRUCTIONS

1. *For *Cashew Ricotta*, soak cashews for at least 4 hours in 1 1/2 cups water. Drain and rinse. Process with basil, white pepper, garlic powder and salt in food processor or bullet blender until smooth. Add water 1 tablespoon at a time as necessary. Set aside.

2. Preheat oven to 350 degrees F. Bring medium pot of lightly salted water to boil. Line square baking pan with parchment, or lightly coat with coconut oil.

3. For *Pasta Sauce*, process all sauce ingredients in food processor or bullet blender, then pour into small pot. Heat over medium heat and stir until warm. Remove from heat and set aside.

4. Slice zucchini into thin wide strips with sharp knife or mandolin. Blanch zucchini sheets in boiling water for about 30 seconds, just to make pliable. Remove and lay on paper towel or parchment. Sprinkle with pinch of salt and pepper.

5. Spread *Pasta Sauce* on zucchini. Place dollop of *Cashew Ricotta* toward one end of zucchini sheet. Roll up zucchini around ricotta until fully rolled.

6. Place rolled zucchini in lined baking sheet and bake for about 15 minutes, until heated through.

7. Remove from oven and serve hot.

Bacon Quesadilla

Quesadillas are good all day long. Kids love them, too! But with cheese and wheat issues—they are totally off the menu for most of us. Not these! With the satisfying flavors of bacon, cilantro, and avocado you won't miss the cheese. And the tortillas are the perfect substitute for the wheat-based original. Make a few and slice and freeze so that you always have a few to pop in the microwave or toaster oven at snack time!

Prep Time: 10 minutes
Cook Time: 20 minutes
Servings: 2

INGREDIENTS

Filling
8 - 12 strips GF bacon

Tortillas
2 tablespoons almond flour
1 1/2 tablespoons coconut flour
1/2 tablespoon flax meal (or ground chia seed)
1/4 cup water
2 eggs
2 tablespoons coconut oil
1/4 teaspoon baking powder
Vegetable oil (for cooking)

Almond Cheese

1 cup skinless almonds*

1/4 cup water

2 tablespoons vegetable oil

1 tablespoon lemon juice

1 tablespoon apple cider vinegar

1 garlic clove

1/2 teaspoon salt

1/4 teaspoon ground white pepper (or black pepper)

Avocado Cream

1 avocado

1/4 cup full-fat coconut cream

Small bunch cilantro

Juice of half lime

INSTRUCTIONS

1. *For *Almond Cheese*, soak almonds in 1 1/2 cups water overnight. Drain and rinse.

2. Add all *Almond Cheese* ingredients to food processor or bullet blender and process until smooth. Add a few extra tablespoons of water if necessary to achieve thick but smooth consistency. Set aside.

3. Preheat oven to 425 degrees F. Heat medium skillet over medium-high heat.

4. Chop bacon and sauté in skillet until crisp and cooked through, about 5 minutes. Remove bacon and set aside.

5. Reserve half of bacon grease. Add small amount of coconut oil to pan.

6. For *Tortillas*, whisk together eggs, vegetable oil and 1/4 cup water in medium bowl. In a separate bowl, blend coconut flour, almond flour, flax or chia seed, and baking powder.

7. Whisk as you slowly pour dry into wet ingredients. If batter appears too thick to spread fairly thin in pan, add up to 4 tablespoons of water 1 tablespoon at a time.

8. Use ladle or dry measure cup to pour 1/2 of batter into hot oiled pan. Tilt pan in circular motion as you pour so batter spreads thinly.

9. Cook batter for about 2 minutes, or until slightly golden and firm. Flip tortilla with tongs or spatula and cook another 2 minutes. Remove and place on paper towel or parchment.

10. Add reserved bacon grease and small amount of vegetable oil to pan. Cook remaining batter for 2 minutes on each side.

11. For *Avocado Cream*, slice avocado in half and pit. Scoop flesh into food processor with coconut cream, lime juice and cilantro. Process until smooth. Transfer to serving dish.

12. To assemble quesadilla, spread *Almond Cheese* over both tortillas. Sprinkle one tortilla with crisp bacon and top with other tortilla.

13. Place quesadilla on sheet pan or baking pan. Bake for 5 minutes.

14. Slice quesadilla with sharp knife or pizza cutter. Serve hot with *Avocado Cream*.

Chicken Taquitos

Here's another Tex-Mex favorite you may have thought you had to give up forever. Not so! Little chicken tacos are a snap to prepare. The chicken is hot and spicy and the cool cheesy layer provides just the right balance. With the homemade salsa, will make you forget that there is anywhere else to get delicious Mexican food this good, this fast! This is another recipe it pays to make in quantity.

Prep Time: 10 minutes
Cook Time: 20 minutes
Servings: 4

INGREDIENTS

Tortillas

2 tablespoons almond flour

1 1/2 tablespoons coconut flour

1/2 tablespoon flax meal (or ground chia seed)

1/4 cup water

2 eggs

2 tablespoons vegetable oil

1/4 teaspoon GF baking powder

Vegetable oil (for cooking)

Almond Cheese

1 cup skinless almonds*

1/4 cup water

2 tablespoons coconut oil

1 tablespoon lemon juice

1 tablespoon apple cider vinegar

1 garlic clove

1/2 teaspoon salt

1/4 teaspoon ground white pepper (or black pepper)

Filling

8 oz chicken

1/2 teaspoon paprika

1/2 teaspoon ground cumin

Salsa

2 plum tomatoes

1/2 small white onion

Small bunch cilantro

1 jalapeño pepper

Squeeze of lime juice

1/2 teaspoon salt

INSTRUCTIONS

1. *For *Almond Cheese*, soak almonds in 1 1/2 cups water overnight. Drain and rinse.

2. Add all *Almond Cheese* ingredients to food processor or bullet blender and process until smooth. Add a few extra tablespoons of water if necessary to achieve thick but smooth consistency. Set aside.

3. Heat medium pan over medium-high heat and coat with vegetable oil. Preheat oven to 400 degrees F.

4. Whisk together eggs, vegetable oil and 1/4 cup water in medium bowl. In a separate bowl, blend coconut flour, almond flour, flax or chia seed, and baking powder.

5. Whisk as you slowly pour dry into wet ingredients. If batter appears too thick to spread fairly thin in pan, add up to 4 tablespoons of water 1 tablespoon at a time.

6. Use ladle or dry measure cup to pour 1/4 of batter into hot oiled pan. Tilt pan in circular motion as you pour so batter spreads thinly.

7. Cook batter for about 2 minutes or until slightly golden and firm. Flip tortilla with tongs or spatula and cook another 2 minutes. Remove and place on paper towel or parchment.

8. Cook remaining batter for 2 minutes on each side. Re-oil pan as necessary.

9. Add 1 tablespoon oil to hot pan.

10. Chop chicken and add to hot oiled pan with paprika and cumin. Sauté about 5 minutes, until golden brown and cooked through.

11. For *Salsa*, finely chop tomato, onion, jalapeño, cilantro and mix with squeeze of lime and salt in serving dish bowl.

12. Spread *Almond Cheese* on tortillas and Place sautéed chicken and salsa down center of each tortilla. Tightly roll each tortilla into long tube and place on sheet pan or baking pan. Pierce wit toothpick to keep roll tight if preferred.

13. Place in oven and bake about 5 - 7 minutes, until just heated through.

14. Remove and serve warm.

Sausage And Peppers

Love, Italian style! Sausage and peppers are a match made in food heaven. A staple of street fairs and festivals, this savory combination can't be beat. For a heartier snack, serve alongside scrambled eggs or a salad. You will understand why people eagerly line up for a plate of this old-world one pot meal.

Prep Time: 5 minutes

Cook Time: 10 minutes

Servings: 4

INGREDIENTS

4 Italian GF sausage links (pork, chicken, etc.)

1 white onion

1 bell pepper

INSTRUCTIONS

1. Heat large skillet over medium heat. Add 1 tablespoon vegetable oil.
2. Peel onion. Stem and seed pepper. Roughly chop onion and pepper. Slice sausage into 3/4 inch slices.
3. Add sausage to hot oiled skillet and sauté about 2 minutes. Then add onion and peppers. Sauté about 8 minutes, until sausage is cooked through and browned.
4. Serve hot.

Baked Sweet Plantains

Goldilocks would have loved this snack! Not too sweet, not too heavy, just right! With the addition of a sprinkle of cinnamon this is comfort food at its best.

Prep Time: 5 minutes

Cook Time: 20 minutes

Servings: 1

INGREDIENTS

1 ripe yellow plantain

1 tablespoon sweetener*

2 tablespoons water

1 teaspoon vegetable oil

1/2 teaspoon ground cinnamon

INSTRUCTIONS

1. Preheat oven to 400 degrees F. Line baking pan with parchment, or lightly coat with vegetable oil.
2. Cut plantain into 3/4 inch slices. Remove peel from each slice.
3. Toss plantains in small bowl with sweetener, water, oil and cinnamon.
4. Arrange plantains in single layer on baking pan. Bake 10 minutes, then turn over and bake another 10 minutes, or until plantains are golden brown and tender.
5. Serve warm.

raw honey or agave nectar

Ants On A Log

Do you remember when you thought that ants at a picnic were fun? Well, the memories will all come back to you when you re-create this classic crowd-pleaser. Still the most fun way to eat celery ever invented!

Prep Time: 5 minutes

Cook Time: 5 minutes

Servings: 2

INGREDIENTS

3 celery stalks

2 tablespoons raisins

Cashew Butter

1 cup cashews

1 teaspoon vegetable oil

1/2 teaspoon ground cinnamon

INSTRUCTIONS

1. Add cashews, cinnamon, and vegetable oil to food processor or bullet blender. Process until smooth. Let mixture rest between periods of processing to reach desired consistency, if necessary.
2. Cut celery stalks into thirds and fill wells with *Cashew Butter*. Place raisins on cashew butter.

3. Serve room temperature. Or refrigerate 10 minutes and serve chilled.

Grilled Pineapple Fruit Salad

Grilling fruit brings a special dimension to the sweet pineapple. With the juiciness of the fruit and the minty accents, this smoky surprise will be a new favorite. It is so easy, yet so sophisticated to serve this as an elegant ending to any meal or as a refreshing light snack.

Prep Time: 5 minutes

Cook Time: 10 minutes

Servings: 4

INGREDIENTS

1/2 pineapple

1 peach

1 cup fresh cherries

1 orange

1 tablespoon fresh mint leaves

Half lemon

INSTRUCTIONS

1. Heat griddle or grill over medium-high heat. Lightly coat with coconut oil.
2. Peel and core pineapple. Cut into half inch slices. Place slice on griddle and grill about 4 - 5 minutes on each side, until grill marks appear and sugars caramelized.
3. Cut peach in half and grill flesh side down for about 5 minutes.

4. Pit cherries and slice in half. Peel orange and cut flesh from white cellulose film and pith.

5. Chop pineapple and peach. Add to medium mixing bowl with cherries and orange wedges. Chiffon mint. Add to bowl and squeeze on lemon juice. Toss to combine.

6. Serve room temperature. Or refrigerate and serve chilled.

Sweet Cinnamon Gluten-Free Pretzel

You know those pretzels at the mall? Yes, the ones that should be declared illegally tempting to those of us on GF diets! Well, these aren't quite the same thing, but they will hold you over in a pinch and the sweet, gooey cinnamon flavor with the luscious coconut cream may take your mind off everything else for a few delightful minutes.

Prep Time: 10 minutes

Cook Time: 20 minutes

Servings: 4

INGREDIENTS

Cinnamon Pretzel

1 cup coconut flour

1/2 cup tapioca flour/starch

1/2 cup vegetable oil

1/2 cup water

2 dried dates

1 egg

2 tablespoon apple cider vinegar

1/2 teaspoon baking soda

1/2 teaspoon GF baking powder

2 teaspoons ground cinnamon

1/2 teaspoon vanilla

1/2 teaspoon ground ginger

1/2 teaspoon salt

Coconut Sweet Cream
1/4 cup full-fat coconut milk
2 tablespoons sweetener
1 tablespoon lemon juice
1/2 teaspoon vanilla

INSTRUCTIONS

1. Preheat oven to 350 degrees F. Heat medium pot over medium-high heat. Line sheet pan with parchment or baking mat.

2. Add dates, vegetable oil, water, vinegar and salt to food processor or bullet blender and process until smooth. Pour mixture into pot. Bring to a boil and remove from heat.

3. Whisk in tapioca flour. Stir with wooden spoon or soft spatula until mixture comes together.

4. Stir in baking soda and baking powder. Continue mixing for a minute. Mixture will foam and expand. Let mixture sit and cool about 5 minutes.

5. Sift in coconut flour and spices. Mix partially, then beat in egg. Mix until combined. Excess coconut flour may sit in bottom of bowl.

6. Turn out dough onto cutting board dusted with any excess coconut flour from mixture. Knead dough for 2 minutes.

7. Cut dough into 4 equal portions. Roll out pieces into ropes and twist to form classic pretzel twist. Pinch together any crumbled dough.

8. Arrange pretzels on lined sheet pan. Brush with coconut oil or full-fat coconut milk.

9. Place sheet pan in oven and bake about 25 minutes, until cooked through.

10. For *Coconut Sweet Cream*, mix coconut milk, vanilla, sweetener and lemon juice with had mixer or whisk until thick and creamy. Transfer to serving dish.

11. Serve pretzels immediately with *Coconut Sweet Cream*. Or allow pretzels to cool and refrigerate sweet cream, and serve chilled.

stevia, raw honey or agave nectar

Blueberry Dumplings

Blueberries are packed with anti-oxidants, which would be enough to rate this yummy treat high on the snack chart. This dish, a lot like a fruit slump or cobbler will amaze you. Try mixing it with other berries or fresh peaches for an endless variety of summer-time pleasures!

Prep Time: 15 minutes

Cook Time: 30 minutes

Servings: 6

INGREDIENTS

Blueberry Filling

2.5 cups blueberries (fresh or frozen)

2 - 4 tablespoons sweetener*

2 tablespoons tapioca flour

Dumplings

1/4 cup coconut flour

3/4 cup almond flour

3 tablespoons cold coconut oil

1 teaspoon baking powder

1/2 teaspoon ground cinnamon

1/2 teaspoon ground ginger

1/4 teaspoon salt

2 eggs

2 tablespoon sweetener

1 teaspoon vanilla

INSTRUCTIONS

1. Sift coconut flour, almond flour, baking powder and salt into small mixing bowl. Add cinnamon and ginger. Cut in cold coconut oil with fork until crumbly. Place in freezer for 10 minutes.
2. Preheat oven to 400 degrees F.
3. Add blueberries and sweetener to medium pot. Heat over medium heat and bring to simmer. Whisk in tapioca flour and simmer about 10 minutes.
4. Pour blueberries into casserole dish and place in hot oven.
5. In medium bowl, beat eggs, sweetener and vanilla. Add chilled flour mixture to eggs and mix until dough comes together.
6. Carefully remove bubbling blueberries from oven and drop 8 dumplings onto berries.
7. Return dish to oven and bake 15 - 20 min, until dumplings are golden, set and cooked through.
8. Remove dish from oven and allow to cool about 5 minutes.
9. Serve warm. Or allow to cool completely and serve room temperature.

*stevia, raw honey or agave nectar

Sweet Papaya Fried Pie

Hand-held pies are a favorite anytime, anywhere! This sweet tropical fruit version puts a whole new twist on regular old pie.

Prep Time: 20 minutes

Cook Time: 20 minutes

Servings: 4

INSTRUCTIONS

Crust

2 cups almond flour

2 eggs

3 tablespoons vegetable oil

1 tablespoon sweetener*

1/4 teaspoon baking soda

1/2 teaspoon ground ginger

1/2 teaspoon salt

Filling

1 cup papaya (cut into chunks)

1 fresh guava (or 1/2 cup guava puree)

2 tablespoons sweetener*

2 tablespoons water

1 teaspoon vanilla

1/2 inch piece fresh ginger

Zest of half lemon

Juice of half lemon

DIRECTIONS

1. For *Crust*, sift almond flour into medium mixing bowl. Add baking soda, ginger and salt.

2. Whisk eggs and sweetener in small mixing bowl, then add to flour and combine. Slowly add coconut oil until formable dough comes together.

3. Roll in plastic wrap or wrap tightly in parchment and refrigerate for 15 minutes.

4. Preheat oven to 400 degrees. Line sheet pan with parchment or baking mat. Cover cutting board with parchment.

5. For *Filling*, peel, pit and dice papaya. Peel and dice ginger. Add papaya and ginger to food processor or bullet blender with sweetener, water, vanilla, lemon juice and zest, and guava puree, or peeled, seeded guava flesh. Process until smooth.

6. Remove dough from refrigerator. Divide dough into 4 portions. Roll dough into balls and flatten on parchment covered cutting board with hands. Roll into circles about 1/8 inch thick with rolling pin.

7. Scoop equal portions of *Filling* into center of one side of dough circle. Fold bare half of dough over filled half. Press edges together, letting any trapped air escape. Crimp edges of dough together with fork. Repeat with remaining dough.

8. Arrange pies on lined sheet pan and bake 15 - 20 minutes, or until dough is golden and cooked through.

9. Serve immediately.

stevia, raw honey or agave nectar

NOTE: Heat large skillet over medium heat , add 1/4 inch coconut oil, and fry pies 2 minutes on each side for traditional *Fried Pies*.

Fried Choco Pie

When only chocolate will do, here's a recipe that will rival all others. The rich, dark, taste of chocolate combines here with the chewy fruit to create an entirely new way to experience everyone's favorite indulgence.

Prep Time: 20 minutes*
Cook Time: 20 minutes
Servings: 4

INSTRUCTIONS

Crust
2 cups almond flour
2 eggs
3 tablespoons vegetable oil
1 tablespoon sweetener*
1/4 teaspoon baking soda
1 tablespoon cocoa powder
1/2 teaspoon ground cinnamon
1/2 teaspoon salt

Filling
1 cup cashews*
1/2 cup dried dates*
1/4 cup coconut cream
3 tablespoons cocoa powder
1 egg

1 teaspoon vanilla

1 teaspoon ground cinnamon

1 teaspoon ground nutmeg

1/2 teaspoon ground black pepper

DIRECTIONS

1. *Soak cashew and dates for at least 4 hours in 2 cups water. Drain, then add all *Filling* ingredients to food processor or bullet blender and process until smooth. Set aside.

2. For *Crust*, sift almond flour into medium mixing bowl. Add baking soda, cocoa, cinnamon and salt.

3. Whisk eggs and sweetener in small mixing bowl, then add to flour and combine. Slowly add vegetable oil until formable dough comes together.

4. Roll in plastic wrap or wrap tightly in parchment and refrigerate for 15 minutes.

5. Preheat oven to 400 degrees. Line sheet pan with parchment or baking mat.

6. Remove dough from refrigerator. Divide dough into 4 portions. Roll dough into balls and flatten on parchment covered cutting board with hands. Roll into circles about 1/8 inch thick with rolling pin.

7. Scoop equal portions of *Filling* into center of one side of dough circle. Fold bare half of dough over filled half. Press edges together, letting any trapped air escape. Crimp edges of dough together with fork. Repeat with remaining dough.

8. Arrange pies on lined sheet pan and bake 15 - 20 minutes, or until dough is golden and cooked through.

9. Serve immediately.

stevia, raw honey or agave nectar

NOTE: Heat large skillet over medium heat , add 1/4 inch vegetable oil, and fry pies 2 minutes on each side for traditional *Fried Pies*.

Chocolate Banana Bites

So easy, you'll wonder why you're not making more of these! They are the perfect treat on hot days and a healthier substitute for ice cream novelties.

Prep Time: 10 minutes

Cook Time: 5 minutes

Servings: 1

INGREDIENTS

1 banana

2 - 4 oz GF bittersweet or semisweet chocolate

3 tablespoons chopped nuts (or flaked coconut)

DIRECTIONS

1. Heat chocolate over double boiler until melted, about 5 minutes.
2. Peel banana and cut in 1 inch slices.
3. Dip banana pieces into chocolate, or spread chocolate over tops of banana slices.
4. Sprinkle nuts or coconut over chocolate.
5. Place dipped, topped bananas in freezer for 5 minutes, or until chocolate is set.
6. Serve chilled.

NOTE: For *Frozen Chocolate Banana Bites*, leave dipped, topped banana pieces in freezer for 20 minutes, then serve.

Fruit 'N Nut Bars

Everyone loves those packaged fruit and nut bars from the grocery store or gym, but they are pricey! Make your own and save! Plus, you can try out your own designer combinations for a really unique bar.

Prep Time: 10 minutes

Cook Time: 10 minutes

Servings: 6

INGREDIENTS

1/4 cup dried cherries

1/2 cup dried apricots

1/4 cup dried cranberries

1/4 cup dried dates

1/3 cup warm water

1 cup cashews

1/2 teaspoon vanilla

1/2 teaspoon ground cinnamon

1/4 teaspoon ground ginger

1/4 teaspoon salt

INSTRUCTIONS

1. Soak dried fruit in warm water for 5 - 10 minutes. Drain and add to food processor or bullet blender with cashews, vanilla, cinnamon, ginger and salt.
2. Process until mixture forms a sticky mass, about 1 minute.

3. Transfer to loaf pan lined with parchment. Fold parchment over mixture and press firmly into bottom of pan with spatula or hand.
4. Refrigerate for 10 minutes. Remove and cut into 6 bars.
5. Serve chilled or room temperature.

Hoppin' Hot Chocolate

Mmmmm. There is nothing like coming inside from a cold winter's day and warming up with a steaming cup of hot chocolate. This one offers every bit of satisfaction as the other, but without the discomfort caused by all that dairy milk. The spicy, exotic twist here of the added cinnamon and other flavors make this a very grown up hot chocolate.

Prep Time: 5 minutes

Cook Time: 15 minutes

Servings: 4

INGREDIENTS

2 cups unsweetened nutmilk (not full-fat coconut milk)

13 oz (1 can) full-fat coconut milk

1/4 cup raw honey or agave nectar

4 oz bittersweet or baking chocolate

2 tablespoons cocoa powder

2 tablespoons instant espresso (or instant coffee)

1 tablespoon ground cinnamon

1 teaspoon vanilla

1 teaspoon ground black pepper

1/2 teaspoon ground cayenne pepper

INSTRUCTIONS

1. Add nutmilk, coconut milk and vanilla to medium pot. Heat over medium-high heat and bring to a boil. Reduce heat and simmer for 10 minutes.

2. Whisk in chocolate, sweetener, cocoa powder, espresso, cinnamon, pepper and cayenne. Whisk occasionally for 5 minutes, until chocolate is melted and mixture becomes thick and creamy.

3. Pour into mugs and serve warm.

Piña Colada Smoothie

Tropical fruit flavors are loved the world over—and this winning combination of coconut and pineapple is the star of the famous rum-based drink. Here, skip the rum, and make this satisfying and nourishing snack part of a healthy and delicious diet! An absolutely perfect summer treat!

Prep Time: 5 minutes

Cook Time: 5 minutes

Servings: 2

INSTRUCTIONS

1 large banana

1 cup pineapple chunks (fresh, frozen or canned)

2 tablespoons flaked coconut

1 cup coconut milk

1 cup ice (crushed preferably)

DIRECTIONS

1. Add banana, pineapple, coconut, coconut milk and ice to high-speed blender. Process until smooth.
2. Pour into chilled glasses and serve immediately.

Bread Recipes

"Corn" Muffins

Prep Time: 5 minutes
Cook Time: 15 minutes
Servings: 12

Wondering what "corn" muffins are? Well, we all know that it's a challenge not being able to eat corn on a gluten-free diet. Here's the answer to that challenge. This recipe is for a lightly sweet golden treat that your family won't be able to resist; and nobody will even miss the corn! Try this quick and easy muffin the next time you're looking for a little something to round out your meal.

INGREDIENTS

1 cup almond flour

2 cage-free eggs

1/4 cup coconut oil

2 tablespoons unsweetened applesauce

1 teaspoon sweetener*

1 teaspoon organic apple cider vinegar

1 teaspoon baking powder

1/2 teaspoon ground turmeric (optional)

Pinch ground white pepper (optional)

INSTRUCTIONS

1. Preheat oven to 350 degrees F. Line muffin pan with paper liners or lightly coat with coconut oil.

2. Beat eggs in medium mixing bowl with hand mixer or whisk until thick and slightly frothy. Add oil, applesauce, sweetener, and vinegar and mix well.

3. Stir in almond meal, baking powder, and turmeric and white pepper (optional) until combined.

4. Use ice cream scoop or tablespoon to scoop batter into muffin pan, about 1/2 - 3/4 full.

5. Bake 15 - 18 minutes until edges are golden brown and the tops are firm.

6. Serve warm or room temperature.

NOTE: Bake in square oiled baking pan for 25 - 35 minutes for **"Corn"** **Bread**.

stevia, raw honey or agave nectar

Gluten-Free English Muffins

Prep Time: 5 minutes

Cook Time: 15 minutes

Servings: 4

These English muffins are so good that I think the Queen would knight them if she could. Make a batch and watch your breakfast table tremble as the hungry stampede emerges from the woodwork. Surprisingly, the English muffin is not a muffin, but a variation of the crumpet which then evolved into a toaster biscuit, thought to be a bit more elegant than a muffin at the time. Enjoy these crumpet style wonders the next time you're hungry for a quick treat.

INGREDIENTS

1/3 cup coconut flour

1/4 cup almond milk (or low-fat coconut milk)

2 tablespoons coconut oil

1 tablespoon unsweetened applesauce

1/2 teaspoon baking soda

1 teaspoon organic apple cider vinegar

Pinch Celtic sea salt

INSTRUCTIONS

1. Preheat oven to 400 degrees F. Coat 4 mini-round cake pans or 4-inch diameter oven safe ramekins with coconut oil.

2. In small mixing bowl mix baking soda and apple cider vinegar together. Set aside and allow to froth.

3. In medium bowl, beat eggs with hand mixer or whisk until thick and frothy. Add flour, milk, applesauce and salt. Combine.

4. Add baking soda and vinegar mixture and blend well until smooth and free of clumps.

5. Pour batter into pans or ramekins and bake for 12 - 15 minutes, until slightly golden and center is firm to the touch.

6. Remove muffins from oven. Loosen from sides of pan or container with knife turn out.

7. Serve warm. Muffins will have traditional **English Crumpet** texture.

NOTE: For crusty, American style **English Muffins**, cut in half and toast in skillet coated with coconut oil. Press muffin down in pan with spatula and flip, browning on both sides.

stevia, raw honey or agave nectar

Skillet Biscuits

Prep Time: 5 minutes

Cook Time: 15 minutes

Servings: 8

Biscuits are the quendisential bread used for stretching a meal, sopping up gravy and holding just about any gooey ingredient safely tucked within. They became popular because they were easy-to-carry and long-lasting foods that easily lent themselves to long journeys. A person could carry a supply of biscuits and add them to any other meat or food they had access to along the way. The longer they baked, the harder they got which in some cases (think of crackers) kept them edible for periods of years. Bake these biscuits to your liking, but a nice soft bite is highly recommended.

INGREDIENTS

2 1/2 cups fine ground almond flour

2 cage-free eggs

1/4 cup coconut oil

1 teaspoon baking soda

1/2 teaspoon Celtic sea salt

1 tablespoon sweetener*

INSTRUCTIONS

1. Preheat oven to 350 degrees F. Line sheet pan with parchment paper.

2. Combine almond flour, baking soda and salt in medium bowl.

3. Separate egg whites into separate medium bowl, and yolk into small bowl. Beat egg whites to soft peaks with hand mixer or whisk.

4. Mix yolks, oil and sweetener into whites. Mix wet ingredients into dry to form soft, solid dough.

5. Roll dough into eight (8)1-inch thick round biscuits with hands. Place on parchment covered sheet pan and bake for 12 - 15 minutes, or until golden and firm on top. Serve warm.

NOTE: Oil square baking pan, gently press in dough, cut into 9 squares, and bake for 20 - 25 minutes for break-away pan biscuits.

stevia, raw honey or agave nectar

Italian Flatbread

Prep Time: 10 minutes

Cook Time: 15 minutes

Servings: 4

Oh no, who stepped on the bread? Flour and water flatbreads baked on a fire-heated rock have been a staple for much of humanity for the past 5,000 years. In Mexico it's the tortilla; for the Scots it is oatcake; in India, chapatti; in China they call it po bin; in Israel, matzoh. The grains may be different but the cooking is remarkably the same. In Italy, it's known as focaccia and the precursor to pizza. The wonderful thing about focaccia is that you can throw almost anything on top of it. Use your imagination and enjoy this simple gluten-free variety either hot or cold.

INGREDIENTS

1 cup coconut flour

1/2 cup tapioca flour

1/4 cup chia seed meal (or flax meal)

2 cage-free eggs

3/4 cup water

1 teaspoon baking powder

1 teaspoon dried basil

1 teaspoon dried oregano

1/2 teaspoon ground black pepper

1/2 teaspoon Celtic sea salt

INSTRUCTIONS

1. Preheat oven to 350 degrees F. Line sheet pan with parchment paper. Prepare two additional sheets of parchment paper.

2. Whisk eggs and water in medium bowl. Set aside.

3. Combine flours, chia meal, baking powder and salt in medium bowl.

4. Pour egg mixture into flour mixture, plus spices. Mix well until dough pulls together. If dough is sticky, add 1 tablespoon of coconut flour at a time to reach proper consistency.

5. Flatten dough into basic square shape with hands on one sheet of parchment on cutting board. Cover with second sheet and use rolling pin flatten dough to about 1/8 inch thick rectangle.

6. Cut flatbread dough with pizza cutter or sharp knife into four equal pieces.

7. Gently remove top used parchment sheet and replace with fresh sheet from sheet pan. Invert sheet pan over dough and flip cutting board and sheet pan over. Replace cutting board and gently remove top used parchment sheet.

8. Use spatula to separate flatbreads. Bake in oven for 12 -15 minutes, until browned and firm. Cool and serve.

NOTE: For crisper **Flatbread**, fry flattened dough segments in oiled skillet over medium heat for about 3 minutes on each side, until puffed and browned.

Indian Naan

Prep Time: 5 minutes

Cook Time: 15 minutes

Servings: 4

Naan is a large leaf- shaped flat bread that is baked, torn and used as a staple accompaniment to hot meals in India. A bit of history; the first known ovens date from the earliest agrarian period (the thousand years or so immediately preceding 3000 BC) and are still used today to make this famous bread. Today, modern manufacturers have essentially made an "easy-bake" version to automate the traditional Tandoor oven. Not to worry though, this recipe is simple and will guide you through how to make your own terrific Naan bread by using just simple ingredients, the stovetop and your favorite skillet.

INGREDIENTS

1/2 cup coconut flour

4 cage-free eggs

1/4 cup coconut oil

1/2 - 2/3 cup water

1/4 tsp baking powder

1/2 teaspoons Celtic sea salt

Coconut oil (for cooking)

INSTRUCTIONS

1. Heat medium skillet over medium-high heat and coat generously with coconut oil.

2. Blend flour, eggs, oil, baking powder, salt and 1/2 cup water in a food processor or bullet blender. Process until smooth. Add liquid if batter is too thick, and coconut flour if too thin. You want a moderately thin batter.

3. Pour 1/4th of batter into hot oiled skillet. Cook until naan bubbles and browns, about 2 minutes. Then flip and cook another 2 minutes, or until golden and firm.

4. Repeat with remaining batter. Re-oil pan as necessary.

5. Drain hot naan on paper towel. Serve warm.

NOTE: For softer **Baked Naan**, bake at 425 degrees F in two (2)9-inch round cake pans generously coated with coconut oil for 10 minutes, or until cooked through.

State Fair Fry Bread

Prep Time: 5 minutes

Cook Time: 15 minutes

Servings: 2

Common now, when is the last time you went to a Native American state fair? Just to put this recipe into context, according to Navajo tradition fry bread was originally made in 1864 using the flour, sugar, salt and lard that was given to them by the United States government when the Navajo Native Americans, were forced to relocate onto land that wouldn't provide the necessary staples of vegetables and beans. Long since, this delicious bread has made it way to becoming a popular item at many state fairs. Now you can make this blue ribbon gluten-free version right in your own kitchen.

INGREDIENTS

1 cup coconut flour

1 cup almond flour (or cashew flour)

1/4 cup tapioca flour/starch

3 cage-free eggs

1/2 cup coconut oil

1/2 cup full-fat coconut milk

1 teaspoon baking powder

2 tablespoons sweetener*

Pinch Celtic sea salt

Water (for thinning)

Coconut oil (for cooking)

INSTRUCTIONS

1. Heat medium skillet over medium-high heat and coat generously with coconut oil.

2. Blend eggs, oil, milk and sweetener in food processor or bullet blender until smooth and a bit airy.

3. In medium bowl, combine flours, baking powder and salt. Add egg mixture and combine to form soft dough. If too tough, add water 1 tablespoon at a time.

4. Form dough into 2 large flat rounds with hands. Place 1 round in pan and cook about 3 minutes, or until puffed and browned. Flip fry bread with tongs or spatula and cook another 3 minutes, or until golden and cooked through.

5. Repeat with remaining dough. Re-oil pan as necessary.

6. Drain hot fry bread on paper towel. Serve warm.

NOTE: For **Baked Fry Bread**, generously coat two 9-inch round cake pans with coconut oil. Press dough into pans and brush tops with coconut oil. Bake at 425 degrees F in for 15 minutes, or until cooked through and golden.

stevia, raw honey or agave nectar

Easy Pocket Pita

Prep Time: 5 minutes

Cook Time: 20 minutes

Servings: 1

Pita bread, or pocket bread as it is sometimes called is a bread of versatility and charm. That's because when it is baking, you can actually watch it puff up like a balloon and then as it cools it flattens. When you slice it and find the pocket inside it's just begging to be filled. No kids, just because it is a pocket, you can't keep old change and frogs in it! Try egg salad, apples and aged cheese, lamb with cucumbers, tomatoes, red lettuce and mint. Oh, the list goes on and so will yours when you bake a fresh pile of pita bread.

INGREDIENTS

1 cup tapioca flour/starch

1 cage-free egg

2 tablespoons coconut oil (or almond oil)

1 teaspoon ground chia seed (flax meal)

5 tablespoons water

1/2 teaspoon baking soda

1/4 teaspoon Celtic sea salt

INSTRUCTIONS

1. Preheat oven to 375 degrees F. Cover sheet pan with parchment paper. Heat small pot over low heat.

2. Mix 1/3 cup flour, chia meal, water and 1 tablespoon oil in pan. Stir until mixture comes together. Remove from heat and cool in freezer.

3. In medium bowl, blend remaining flour, baking soda and salt. Then add egg and remaining oil. Mix until combined.

4. Add cooled chia mixture to bowl. Mix to combine, then remove and knead to form dough.

5. Form round disk, then flatten on baking sheet lined with parchment.

6. Bake about 15 minutes. Carefully turn over with spatula and bake another 5 - 10 minutes, or until crisp.

7. Remove from oven and cut into wedges. Serve warm or cooled.

NOTE: For **Pita Chips** , place baked wedges on oiled sheet pan, brush tops with coconut oil and broil in oven for about 2 minutes on each side. *Watch carefully and do not burn!*

Frontier Tortillas

Prep Time: 5 minutes

Cook Time: 10 minutes

Servings: 2

A tortilla is a Mexican version of flatbread you can use in a multitude of ways. Use them for tacos, burritos, as a wrap or enjoy eating them warm just by themselves. Flatbread tortillas have been eaten for thousands of years northern Mexico, where they remain a staple. Made the traditional way, with corn and/or wheat flour they do not fit into a gluten-free diet. Our fantastic version does and we think you'll find tortillas as fun to make as they are to eat.

INGREDIENTS

2 tablespoons almond flour

1 1/2 tablespoons coconut flour

1/2 tablespoon flax meal (or ground chia seed)

2 cage-free eggs

1/4 cup water

2 tablespoons coconut oil

1/4 teaspoon baking powder

Extra water

Coconut oil (for cooking)

INSTRUCTIONS

1. Heat medium frying pan over medium-high heat and coat with coconut oil.

2. Whisk together eggs, coconut oil and 1/4 cup water in medium bowl. In a separate bowl, blend coconut flour, almond flour, flax or chia seed, and baking powder.

3. Slowly whisk as you pour dry into wet ingredients. If batter appears too thick to spread fairly thin in pan, add water 1 tablespoon at a time. Do not exceed 4 tablespoons.

4. Use ladle or dry measure cup to pour 1/2 of batter into hot oiled pan. Tilt pan in circular motion as you pour so batter spreads thinly.

5. Cook batter for about 2 minutes or until slightly golden and firm. Flip tortilla with tongs or spatula and cook another 2 minutes. Remove and place on paper towel or parchment.

6. Cook remaining batter for 2 minutes on each side. Re-oil pan as necessary.

7. Fill warm tortillas with meat or veggies of choice and serve warm.

Coconut Crisps

Prep Time: 10 minutes

Cook Time: 10 minutes

Servings: 4

Looking for something to satisfy your crunch craving? Yes, crunch craving; you know that time of day when you just need something extra crunchy to munch on. This is it! Coconut Crisps are light, sweet treats that are a lot of fun to bake and even more fun to eat. Did you know that every bit of the coconut can be used? As a result, coconuts are called the "Tree of Life". So why not make good use of one yourself and bake up a quick batch of yummy Coconut Crisps?

INGREDIENTS

1 cup coconut flour

3/4 cup almond flour

4 cage-free egg whites

1/4 cup coconut oil

1/4 cup coconut crème

1/4 cup sweetener

1/2 cup flaked coconut

1 teaspoon vanilla

1/2 teaspoon baking soda

3/4 teaspoon Celtic sea salt

1/2 teaspoon ground white pepper (or black pepper)

INSTRUCTIONS

1. Preheat oven to 375 degrees F. Line sheet pan with parchment paper or coat with coconut oil. Prepare two additional sheets of parchment.

2. Whisk egg and oil with hand mixer or whisk until blended and slightly frothy. Add sweetener, coconut crème and vanilla, and continue blending.

3. Sift in half of flour, baking soda, vanilla, salt and pepper. Add coconut flakes. Sift in remaining flour. Stir and bring dough together.

4. Form dough into rectangle and flatten with hands on parchment. Cover with second sheet of parchment and flatten to about 1/4 inch with rolling pin. Remove top layer of parchment.

5. Cut rectangles from dough with pizza cutter or sharp knife. Carefully flip dough onto sheet pan. Arrange at least 1/2 inch apart on sheet pan.

6. Bake for about 10 minutes, or until crisp and golden brown. Remove and let cool. Serve room temperature.

Strawberry Bread

Prep Time: 10 minutes

Cook Time: 10 minutes

Servings: 12 - 16

Remember that old Beatles song Strawberry Bread forever? Oops, that wasn't it, but it should have been; this bread deserves its own fan club. Fresh ripe strawberries combine perfectly in this moist flavorful bread highlighted with hints of spicy ginger and pepper. Enjoy the sweet fragrance as it wafts through your home as Strawberry Bread bakes. Once in a while a recipe is so good that you know it's going to be a hit for years to come and this is one of them.

INGREDIENTS

1 cup coconut flour

3/4 cup cashew flour (or almond flour)

1/4 cup ground chia seed (or flax meal)

1/2 cup coconut oil

2 cage-free eggs

1/4 cup coconut crème

1/4 cup sweetener*

1/4 cup unsweetened apple sauce

1 teaspoons baking powder

1 tablespoon ground cinnamon

1 teaspoon ground ginger

1 teaspoon ground white pepper (or black pepper)

1 teaspoon Celtic sea salt

2 cups fresh sliced strawberries

1/2 cup chopped walnuts (optional)

INSTRUCTIONS

1. Preheat oven to 350 degrees F. Line muffin pan with paper liners or coat with coconut oil.

2. In large bowl, whisk eggs with hand mixer or whisk until frothy and light. Add coconut oil, sweetener and applesauce. Blend until combined. Slice strawberries, and fold in with walnuts (optional).

3. In medium bowl, blend flours, chia meal, baking powder, salt and spices. Stir flour blend into strawberry mixture until well combined.

4. Use ice cream scoop or tablespoon to scoop equal portions of batter into muffin pans, 1/2 - 3/4 full. Line or oil more muffin pans if excess batter remains.

5. Bake for 15 minutes, or until golden brown and firm but springy to the touch.

6. Cool enough to handle. Serve warm or room temperature.

NOTE: Bake in square oiled baking pan for 25 - 35 minutes or two oiled loaf pans for 35 - 45 minutes for **Strawberry Loaves**.

stevia, raw honey or agave nectar

Primal Apple Cider Bread

Prep Time: 10 minutes
Cook Time: 20 minutes
Servings: 24

Imagine, your back in primitive times; a caveman is walking along and sees an apple tree. Under the tree are fallen apples, so he picks one up. It kind of soft and old looking but he takes a bite anyway. Hmm..it tastes pretty good, but sour. I'll take this back to woman and she cook. Hence, many thousands of years later comes our recipe for Primal Apple Cider Bread. That was one smart woman and we hope that you'll enjoy this bread as much as our caveman friend did. Happy baking!

INGREDIENTS

2 cups coconut flour

1 cup almond flour

12 ounces organic hard cider

2 cage-free eggs

1/2 cup unsweetened applesauce

1 tart apple

2 tablespoons baking powder

1 teaspoon ground nutmeg

1 teaspoon ground black pepper

1 teaspoon Celtic sea salt

INSTRUCTIONS

1. Preheat oven to 375 degrees F. Line 2 muffin pans with paper liners or coat with coconut oil.

2. Peel, core and grate or dice apple, and place in large bowl. Pour hard apple cider over apples, plus nutmeg and black pepper.

3. In medium bowl, whisk eggs with hand mixer or whisk until frothy and light. Add applesauce and blend until combined. Add egg mixture to cider and apples.

4. Slowly sift and stir flours, baking powder and salt into wet ingredients.

5. Use ice cream scoop or tablespoon to scoop equal portions of batter into muffin pans, 1/2 - 3/4 full.

6. Bake for 15 - 20 minutes, or until golden brown and firm but springy to the touch.

7. Cool enough to handle. Serve warm or room temperature.

NOTE: Bake in square oiled baking pan for 35 - 45 minutes or two oiled loaf pans for 45 - 55 minutes for **Primal Apple Cider Loaves**.

*stevia, raw honey or agave nectar

Pumpkin Coconut Bread

Prep Time: 5 minutes

Cook Time: 25 minutes

Servings: 12

After trying a slice of this bread, you won't have to wonder why The Great Pumpkin makes very few appearances on the cartoon Peanuts. The whole town would be hunting it down just to have a chance of mass producing this recipe. It's not often that a new idea comes along to update an old favorite like this. The addition of coconut gives it a delicious chew and the addition of pumpkin seeds is ingenious. It'll leave you wondering, why didn't I think of that?

INGREDIENTS

1 3/4 cups coconut flour

2 cage-free eggs

1/4 cup coconut oil

1/2 coconut milk

1/2 unsweetened applesauce

1/4 cup sweetener*

15 oz (1 can) pumpkin puree

2 teaspoons baking soda

1 tablespoon ground cinnamon

1 teaspoon ground nutmeg

1 teaspoon Celtic sea salt

1/2 cup flaked coconut

1/4 cup pumpkin seeds

Water

INSTRUCTIONS

1. Preheat oven to 350 degrees F. Coat square baking pan with coconut oil.

2. Process eggs, coconut oil, coconut milk, applesauce and sweetener in food processor or blender until thick and lightened. Pour into medium mixing bowl. Mix in pumpkin puree and spices.

3. Mix in flour, baking soda, flaked coconut and pumpkin seeds. Stir until combined.

4. Pour batter into oiled baking pan. Bake 20 - 25 minutes, or until firm but springy in center.

5. Serve warm or room temperature.

NOTE: Bake in lined or oiled muffin pan for 15 - 20 minutes for **Pumpkin Coconut Muffins**.

stevia, raw honey or agave nectar

Avocado Spice Bread

Prep Time: 5 minutes

Cook Time: 20 minutes

Servings: 12

Everybody loves good spice bread and you won't believe how luscious the addition of creamy avocado makes this one. Did you know that the avocado is a fruit and not a vegetable! It is actually a member of the berry family. Who'd a thunk? Back in the day, the avocado had an infamous reputation; it was said to be an aphrodisiac and anyone who purchased or ate one was asking for some slanderous assault. We say, bahh! Enjoy avocados every chance you get and in every way you can. They're delicious and healthy, so make this sumptuous Avocado Spice Bread and happily observe the smiles on the faces of loved ones when they bite in. It'll be your little secret.

INGREDIENTS

1 3/4 cups almond flour

1/4 cup flax seed meal (or ground chia seed)

3 cage-free eggs

3 avocados

1/2 cup unsweetened applesauce (or apple butter)

1/4 cup sweetener*

1/2 cup fresh squeezed orange juice

1 tablespoon orange zest

1 tablespoon baking powder

1 teaspoon ground cinnamon

1 teaspoon ground allspice

1 teaspoon ground black pepper

1 teaspoon Celtic sea salt

INSTRUCTIONS

1. Preheat oven to 350 degrees F. Coat square baking pan with coconut oil.
2. Slice avocados in half, pit, and scoop flesh into food processor or blender. Add eggs, applesauce, sweetener and orange juice and blend until smooth.
3. Pour avocado blend into medium mixing bowl. Stir in almond flour, flax meal, baking powder, salt, orange zest and spices until combined.
4. Pour batter into oiled baking pan. Bake 20 - 25 minutes, or until firm but springy in center.
5. Serve warm or room temperature.

NOTE: Bake in lined or oiled muffin pan for 15 - 20 minutes for **Avocado Spice Muffins**.

stevia, raw honey or agave nectar

Cocoa Bread

Prep Time: 10 minutes
Cook Time: 20 minutes
Servings: 8

Cocoa, used throughout history as a folk medicine, just happens to be one of the most delicious ingredients in this recipe for this puffy chocolaty bread. According to a recent Harvard study, flavonoid-rich cocoa consumption is associated with decreased blood pressure, improved blood vessel health, and improvement in cholesterol levels. That's good enough for me! Enjoy good eats and feel good too. Make some delectable Cocoa bread in the form of muffins, or if you're feeling decadent an entire loaf and share it with friends. It'll go fast, but the delicious memories will last a long, long time.

INGREDIENTS

1 cup coconut flour

6 cage-free eggs

1/2 cup unsweetened applesauce

1/4 cup coconut milk

1/2 teaspoon baking soda

2 tablespoons raw cocoa powder

1/2 teaspoon ground black pepper

1/2 teaspoon salt

INSTRUCTIONS

1. Preheat oven to 350 degrees F. Coat 2 small loaf pans with coconut oil.

2. Separate eggs. In large bowl, whisk egg whites to soft peaks with hand mixer or whisk. Add yolks, applesauce and coconut milk. Mix until combined.

3. Sift in flour, baking soda, cocoa powder, black pepper and salt. Stir to combine.

4. Pour batter into oiled loaf pans. Bake 20 - 25 minutes, or until firm but springy in center.

5. Serve warm or room temperature.

NOTE: Bake in large oiled loaf pan for 30 - 40 minutes for **GF Cocoa Loaf**.

Grain-Free Gingerbread

Prep Time: 5 minutes

Cook Time: 20 minutes

Servings: 8

Yum, gingerbread!!! Remember warm, spicy gingerbread right out of the oven? That's one of my childhood favorites and now you can make some warm memories for someone too. The juice from ginger roots is often used as a spice in Indian recipes, and is a quintessential ingredient of Chinese, Korean, Japanese and many South Asian cuisines for flavoring. Our recipe for a gluten-free version is full of applesauce, cinnamon and ginger juice flavor and is absolutely scrumptious.

INGREDIENTS

2 cups almond flour

2 tablespoons ground chia seed (or flax meal)

2 cage-free eggs

1/2 cup unsweetened applesauce

1/4 cup coconut oil

1/4 cup sweetener*

1 tablespoon baking powder

1 teaspoon baking soda

2 tablespoons ground ginger

1 tablespoon vanilla

1 tablespoon ground cinnamon

1 teaspoon ground black pepper

1/2 teaspoon ground cloves

1/2 teaspoon cardamom (optional)

1 oz fresh ginger juice (optional)

INSTRUCTIONS

1. Preheat oven to 350 degrees F. Coat 2 small loaf pans with coconut oil.

2. In large bowl, beat eggs until light and thickened. Add applesauce, oil, sweetener and ginger juice (optional). Beat well.

3. In medium bowl, blend all dry ingredients well. Slowly stir flour mixture into egg mixture.

4. Pour batter into loaf pans and bake for 20 - 25 minutes, or until toothpick inserted into center comes out clean.

5. Let cool slightly. Insert knife around edges and remove from pan. Serve warm or room temperature.

NOTE: Bake in large oiled loaf pan for 35 - 45 minutes for **Grain-Free Gingerbread Loaf**.

raw honey, agave nectar, grade B maple syrup, molasses

Citrus Curry Spice Bread

Prep Time: 5 minutes

Cook Time: 20 minutes

Servings: 8

Both citrus and curry are known for their spicy and zesty combination and are used in many savory dishes throughout the Middle East. We've taken this successful duo a step further and created Citrus Curry Bread. This bread is unique in that it has enough body to be eaten and enjoyed alongside savory dishes as well as just enough sweetness to be served as a scrumptious dessert. Try it on the side of your next seafood dish or afterward topped with a nice dollop of freshly made gluten-free whipped cream. Top it off with a little candied ginger; Your guests will thank you.

INGREDIENTS

2 cups almond flour

2 cage-free eggs

1/2 cup unsweetened applesauce

1/4 cup coconut oil

Juice of 1 lemon

Juice of 1 orange

1 teaspoon lemon zest

1 teaspoon orange zest

1 tablespoon apple cider vinegar

2 tablespoons baking powder

1 tablespoon vanilla

1 tablespoon curry powder

1 teaspoon ground cinnamon

1 teaspoon ground ginger

1 teaspoon ground white pepper (or black pepper)

1 teaspoon cardamom (optional)

1/ 4 cup pumpkin seeds (optional)

Pinch Celtic sea salt

INSTRUCTIONS

1. Preheat oven to 350 degrees F. Coat 2 small loaf pans with coconut oil.

2. Separate eggs. In large bowl, whisk egg whites to soft peaks with hand mixer or whisk. Add yolks, applesauce, oil, juices, zests and vinegar. Beat well.

3. In medium bowl, blend flour, baking powder, spices and salt. Stir flour mixture into egg mixture.

4. Pour batter into loaf pans and bake for 20 - 25 minutes, or until toothpick inserted into center comes out clean.

5. Let cool slightly. Insert knife around edges and remove from pan. Serve warm or room temperature.

NOTE: Bake in large oiled loaf pan for 35 - 45 minutes for **Citrus Curry Spice Loaf**.

stevia, raw honey or agave nectar

Banana Nut Bread

Prep Time: 5 minutes

Cook Time: 20 minutes

Servings: 9

Raise your hand if you love Banana Nut Bread! Go ahead, it's o.k., I'll wait. Now take a look at our gluten-free recipe for one that will outdo them all. Grandma used to say, ""make sure that your bananas are black-ripe." She's chide me if I used any that weren't just because "they just won't taste right!" Well, I've grown to cherish that advice and pass it on to you. So the next time a couple of those bananas are looking pretty paltry, don't throw them into anything but this bread; and don't forget to thank grandma.

INGREDIENTS

3/4 cup of almond flour

1/4 cup of coconut flour

2 tablespoons flax meal (or ground chia seed)

2 cage-free eggs

2 overripe bananas

1/4 sweetener*

2 tablespoons coconut oil

1/4 cup walnuts

1/4 cup hazelnuts

1 tablespoon baking powder

1 tablespoon cinnamon

1 teaspoon nutmeg

1 teaspoon vanilla

1/2 teaspoon Celtic sea salt

INSTRUCTIONS

1. Preheat oven to 350 degrees F. Coat square baking pan with coconut oil.

2. In medium bowl, beat eggs, bananas, oil, flax or chia, and sweetener.

3. In separate bowl, blend flour, baking powder, salt and spices. Pour banana mixture in flour mixture and blend. Fold in nuts.

4. Pour batter into baking pan and bake for 20 - 25 minutes, or until browned and firm in the center.

5. Let cool slightly. Serve warm or room temperature.

NOTE: Bake in oiled loaf pan for 35 - 45 minutes for **Banana Nut Loaf**.

stevia, raw honey or agave nectar

Simple Squash Muffins

Prep Time: 10 minutes

Cook Time: 15 minutes

Servings: 12

You've all heard of squash. There's the game and then there's the vegetable; just to clear up any confusion, that's the one were talking about here. Historically, squash was one of the "Three Sisters" planted by Native Americans. The Three Sisters were the three main native crop plants: maize (corn), beans, and squash. When planted together, the cornstalk provided support for the climbing beans, and shade for the squash. Sounds very wise and so is this recipe custom made to be both gluten-free and a mouth watering way to put that squash to good use.

INGREDIENTS

1 1/2 cups almond flour

2 tablespoons tapioca flour/starch

2 cage-free eggs

1 1/2 cups grated squash (zucchini, acorn squash, summer squash, etc.)

1/4 cup coconut oil

1/2 cup unsweetened applesauce

1/4 cup sweetener

1/2 cup walnuts

1 teaspoon baking soda

1 teaspoon baking powder

1 tablespoon ground cinnamon

1 teaspoon vanilla

1/2 teaspoon Celtic sea salt

INSTRUCTIONS

1. Preheat oven to 350 degrees F. Line muffin pan with paper liners or coconut oil.
2. Peel and chop squash. Process walnuts in food processor or bullet blender until coarsely ground. Add squash, eggs, oil, applesauce and sweetener to food processor or blender with and process until mixture is blended but slightly chunky.
3. In medium bowl, blend flours, baking soda and powder, spices and salt. Pour squash mixture into flour mixture and combine.
4. Use ice cream scoop or tablespoon to scoop batter into muffin tins, about 1/2 - 3/4 full.
5. Bake 15 - 18 minutes until muffins are golden brown and tops are firm to the touch.
6. Serve warm or room temperature.

NOTE: Bake in oiled loaf pan for 35 - 45 minutes for **Simple Squash Loaf**.

stevia, raw honey or agave nectar

Sunshine Muffins

Prep Time: 10 minutes
Cook Time: 15 minutes
Servings: 12

What a nice way to start your day! Muffins made with ingredients like apple, orange, carrot and ginger just have to be dynamite. You won't be fortunate enough to find these gluten-free Sunshine muffins at your local bakery; after your friends are asking for more you just may have to open one yourself. Enjoy these treats with a nice cup of steaming hot coffee and you can't go wrong. Don't forget the children; these make a great lunch box treat as well.

INGREDIENTS

1 1/2 cups almond flour

2 cage-free eggs

1 1/2 cups grated carrot

1/4 cup coconut oil

1/4 cup unsweetened applesauce

1/2 cup fresh squeezed orange juice

1 tablespoon orange zest

1 tablespoon grated fresh ginger

1 tablespoon ground ginger

1 teaspoon vanilla

1 teaspoon baking soda

1 teaspoon baking powder

1/2 teaspoon Celtic sea salt

INSTRUCTIONS

1. Preheat oven to 350 degrees F. Line muffin pan with paper liners or coconut oil.

2. Peel ginger. Grate ginger and carrots. In medium bowl beat eggs with hand mixer or whisk until light and a bit frothy. Add oil, applesauce, orange juice and zest. Beat well. Fold in carrots and ginger.

3. Sift and stir in flour, baking soda and powder, spices and salt until combined.

4. Use ice cream scoop or tablespoon to scoop batter into muffin tins, about 1/2 - 3/4 full.

5. Bake 15 - 18 minutes, or until toothpick inserted into center comes out clean.

6. Serve warm or room temperature.

NOTE: Bake in oiled loaf pan for 35 - 45 minutes for **Sunshine Bread**.

Cranberry Pistachio Scones

Prep Time: 10 minutes
Cook Time: 25 minutes
Servings: 8

It might surprise you that scones are not actually a pastry, they are considered a single serving cake or bread. Usually made round if store-bought, when prepared at home, they take various shapes including triangles, rounds and squares. We say, have fun and make them into stars if you'd like. Our Cranberry Pistachio Scones may be called single serving, but they are so good that it may be hard to stop at just one. Enjoy them along with a traditional cup of tea or any time you just feel like a lightly sweet and nutty treat.

INGREDIENTS

2 cups almond flour

1/3 cup arrowroot flour

1 cage-free egg

1/4 cup organic coconut oil

2 tablespoons liquid sweetener*

2 teaspoons baking powder

1/2 teaspoon vanilla

1/2 teaspoon Celtic sea salt

1/4 cup pistachio nuts

1/4 cup dried cranberries

INSTRUCTIONS

1. Preheat oven to 350 degrees F. Line sheet pan with parchment or coat with coconut oil.

2. Whisk together flours, baking powder, salt and vanilla in large mixing bowl.

3. In small mixing bowl, combine egg, oil and sweetener with hand mixer or whisk. Beat briskly while slowly pouring in coconut oil.

4. Add egg mixture to flour blend and mix until well combined.

5. Fold in cranberries and pistachios until incorporated. Form dough into ball and place on sheet pan . Pat down to flatten to about 1/2 inch thick circle.

6. Cut into eight wedges with pizza cutter or sharp knife. Arrange at least 1 inch apart on sheet pan and bake for 20 - 25 minutes , or until edges are golden brown.

7. Remove and cool. Serve room temperature.

fresh squeezed orange juice, raw honey, agave nectar or grade B maple syrup

Sweet Potato Basil Rolls

Prep Time: 10 minutes

Cook Time: 20 minutes

Servings: 6

Divine is the word that comes to mind when I think of Sweet Potato Basil Rolls. You couldn't beat this combination with a bat! Sweet potatoes have long been known for their somewhat starchy yet sweet flavor; matched up with zingy, spicy basil as an undertone and you couldn't ask for a more delightful and flavorful roll or loaf of bread. Serve these at dinnertime, but make sure to keep this recipe handy for special occasions.

INGREDIENTS

1 cup tapioca flour/starch

1/4 - 1/3 cup coconut flour

1 cage-free egg

1/3 cup warm water

1/4 cup coconut oil

1/2 cup organic canned yams

1 teaspoon baking soda

1 teaspoon apple cider vinegar

Medium bunch fresh basil leaves

1 teaspoon rosemary

1/2 teaspoon ground white pepper (or black pepper)

1 teaspoon Celtic sea salt

INSTRUCTIONS

1. Preheat oven to 350 degrees F. Line sheet pan with parchment paper or coat with coconut oil.

2. Whisk egg in small bowl. Chop basil and rosemary. Whisk yams, vinegar and herbs into egg.

3. In medium bowl, blend tapioca flour, 1/4 cup coconut flour, baking powder, salt and pepper. Stir in warm water and oil. Add sweet potato mixture and mix until well combined.

4. If necessary, add coconut flour or water 1 tablespoon at a time to form soft and slightly sticky dough.

5. Use ice cream scoop or large spoon to scoop out 6 portions of dough and roll into round or oblong balls. Dust hands with extra tapioca flour to prevent sticking.

6. Place rolls on sheet pan and pat down slightly. Bake 20 minutes, or until edges are golden brown and tops are firm. Serve warm or room temperature.

NOTE: For **Sweet Potato Basil French Bread**, roll dough into single log and bake at 325 degrees F for 30 - 35 minutes, or until outside is toasted and center is cooked through.

Garlic 'N Herb Rolls

Prep Time: 10 minutes

Cook Time: 20 minutes

Servings: 6

When I think of garlic, I think of love. It's always a happy thing when the one you love eats garlic when you do, don't you think? Otherwise, no kissing; that's for sure. All kidding aside, these Garlic and Herb Rolls are terrific. Garlic is such a wonderful plant and healthful in many ways. Did you know that it is actually a close relative to an onion? It's know to help prevent heart disease as well as many other ailments. Even Hippocrates mentioned it for keeping away unwanted bugs; how about that? Add fresh rosemary, parsley marjoram and basil and you've got yourself a delectable mouthful. You'll find yourself making double batches.

INGREDIENTS

1 cup tapioca flour/starch

1/4 - 1/3 cup coconut flour

1 cage-free egg

1/2 cup warm water

1/4 cup coconut oil

1/4 cup unsweetened applesauce

1/2 teaspoon baking soda

1 teaspoon apple cider vinegar

2 garlic cloves

Small bunch fresh basil

1 teaspoon dried parsley

1 teaspoon rosemary

Small pinch fresh marjoram (optional)

1/2 teaspoon ground black pepper

1 teaspoon Celtic sea salt

INSTRUCTIONS

1. Preheat oven to 350 degrees F. Line sheet pan with parchment paper or coat with coconut oil.

2. Whisk egg in small bowl. Peel and mince garlic, plus rosemary, fresh basil and marjoram (optional). Whisk applesauce, vinegar, garlic and fresh herbs into egg.

3. In medium bowl, blend tapioca flour, 1/4 cup coconut flour, baking soda, salt and dried spices. Stir in warm water and oil. Add egg mixture and mix until well combined.

4. If necessary, add coconut flour or water 1 tablespoon at a time to form soft and slightly sticky dough.

5. Use ice cream scoop or large spoon to scoop out 6 portions of dough and roll into round or oblong balls. Dust hands with extra tapioca flour to prevent sticking.

6. Place rolls on sheet pan and pat down slightly. Bake 20 minutes, or until edges are golden brown and tops are firm. Serve warm or room temperature.

NOTE: For **Garlic 'N Herb Italian Bread**, roll dough into single log and bake at 325 degrees F for 30 - 35 minutes, or until outside is toasted and center is cooked through.

Savory Tomato Rolls

Prep Time: 10 minutes

Cook Time: 20 minutes

Servings: 6

Roll making can be so much fun; get the group involved. When you get a chance, take a look at all of the shapes you can make and get creative. Just have fun with this wonderful dough and enjoy the savory results. Tomato and herbs are a natural combination and go well with such a variety of dishes. Try these to jazz up your next barbecue along with a stack of freshly slices tomatoes on the side. They're a real crowd pleaser.

INGREDIENTS

1 cup tapioca flour/starch

1/4 - 1/3 cup coconut flour

1 cage-free egg

1/2 cup warm organic tomato sauce

1/4 cup coconut oil

1/4 cup fresh tomato puree (or minced tomato flesh, no skin)

1/2 teaspoon baking soda

1 teaspoon apple cider vinegar

1 teaspoon dried basil

1 teaspoon dried oregano

1/2 teaspoon ground black pepper

1/2 teaspoon Celtic sea salt

INSTRUCTIONS

1. Preheat oven to 350 degrees F. Line sheet pan with parchment paper or coat with coconut oil.

2. Process fresh skinned tomato flesh in food processor or bullet blender. Or mince. Whisk egg in small bowl. Whisk in fresh tomato and vinegar.

3. In medium bowl, blend tapioca flour, 1/4 cup coconut flour, baking soda, salt and spices. Stir in warm tomato sauce and oil. Add egg mixture and mix until well combined.

4. If necessary, add coconut flour or water 1 tablespoon at a time to form soft and slightly sticky dough.

5. Use ice cream scoop or large spoon to scoop out 6 portions of dough and roll into round or oblong balls. Dust hands with extra tapioca flour to prevent sticking.

6. Place rolls on sheet pan and pat down slightly. Bake 20 minutes, or until edges are golden brown and tops are firm. Serve warm or room temperature.

NOTE: For **Savory Tomato French Bread**, roll dough into single long log and bake at 325 degrees F for 30 - 35 minutes, or until outside is toasted and center is cooked through.

Sage Sausage Buns

Prep Time: 10 minutes

Cook Time: 15 minutes

Servings: 8

Sage and sausage make me think of stuffing and the wonderful meals that go with it. These rolls take those memories, some of which are holidays, into a zone that can be enjoyed every day. When is the last time you had meat baked right into your bread? It's not typically how you would think of sausage and eggs, is it? With this recipe, you'll discover the goodness of extra special ingredients every time you take a savory bite. Gluten free eating can be oh so good.

INGREDIENTS

8 oz uncooked natural sage sausage

3/4 cup coconut flour

4 cage-free eggs

1/4 cup unsweetened applesauce

1/4 almond milk

1 teaspoon baking powder

2 tablespoons ground sage

1 tablespoon fresh basil

1 teaspoon ground white pepper (or black pepper)

1/2 teaspoon salt

INSTRUCTIONS

1. Preheat oven to 350 degrees F. Coat muffin pan with coconut oil. Heat medium skillet over medium heat.

2. Brown sausage in skillet for about 5 minutes, until half way cooked. Set aside and reserve leftover oil.

3. While sausage browns, separate eggs. In large bowl, whisk egg whites to soft peaks with hand mixer or whisk. Add yolks, applesauce and almond milk. Mix until combined.

4. Mince basil. Sift flour, baking soda and salt into egg mixture. Add pepper, sage and basil. Stir to combine.

5. Distribute par-cooked sausage evenly into each muffin pan cup. Use ice cream scoop or spoon to scoop batter on top of sausage. Fill each cup no more than 3/4 full.

6. Baste with sausage dripping before placing in oven. Bake 15 - 20 minutes, or until tops are golden brown and firm to the touch.

7. Turn out buns onto plate. Serve warm or room temperature.

NOTE: Bake in oiled square baking pan for 30 - 40 minutes for **Sage Sausage Bread**.

New Yorkshire Puddings

Prep Time: 10 minutes

Cook Time:30 minutes

Servings: 12

Yorkshire pudding is one of Britain's favorites. For the longest time I wondered about why pudding was so popular and special. It turns out that Yorkshire Pudding is not the creamy sweet concoction we think of, it is a batter pudding. Fresh from the oven it should be golden brown with a crisp on the outside and soft middle. This New Yorkshire Pudding is quick, easy to make and with this, our gluten free recipe, it's sure to be a stand-by every time you make a roast.

INGREDIENTS

2 cage-free eggs

1/2 cup coconut milk

1/4 cup almond flour

1/4 cup arrowroot flour

1/4 cup hazelnut flour (walnut flour or cashew flour)

1 tablespoons coconut flour

1/2 teaspoon baking soda

Pinch Celtic sea salt

Coconut oil (for cooking)

INSTRUCTIONS

1. Preheat oven to 400 degrees F. Line muffin pan with paper liners or pour 1/2 teaspoon coconut oil into each cup and place muffin pan in oven.

2. In medium bowl, beat eggs, milk and salt. Add flours and baking soda. Mix well. Set aside for 5 minutes while batter thickens to pudding consistency.

3. Once thickened, carefully remove hot muffin pan, and use ice cream scoop or spoon to pour batter into cups. Bake 5 minutes.

4. Reduce heat to 350 degrees F and bake 20 - 25 minutes, or until puffed and golden.

5. Turn out and plate. Serve Warm.

Baking Recipes

Coconut Macaroons

Prep Time: 10 minutes

Cook Time: 20 minutes

Servings: 12

Simply perfect! Easy, quick, and packed with the delicious flavors of vanilla and coconut, you can whip up a batch of these sweet treats any time you crave a little something.

INGREDIENTS

6 egg whites

3 cups flaked coconut

1/2 cup sweetener*

1 tablespoon coconut oil

1 teaspoon vanilla

1/4 teaspoon salt

INSTRUCTIONS

1. Preheat oven to 350 degrees F. Line a sheet pan with parchment paper or baking mat.
2. In large mixing bowl, beat room temperature egg whites with hand mixer to stiff peaks, about 7 - 8 minutes.
3. Beat in sweetener, vanilla and salt until combined. Fold in 1 cup of coconut at a time.
4. Use ice cream scoop or spoon to drop rounds of batter onto prepared sheet pan.

5. Bake for about 20 minutes, or until coconut is toasted and browned.

6. Allow to cool on pan for 10 minutes. Then remove from pan.

7. Serve warm. Or allow to cool completely and serve room temperature.

raw honey or agave nectar

Blackberry Dumplings

Prep Time: 15 minutes

Cook Time: 20 minutes

Servings: 8

Whether you know them as blackberries, brambleberries, dewberries, or thimbleberries , you know that these little fruits are bursting with color and flavor. You might not know that they are loaded with antioxidants and vitamin C as well. I can't think of a yummier way to enjoy them than in this sweet and crumbly baked dish.

INGREDIENTS

Blackberry Filling

2 1/2 cups blackberries (fresh or frozen)

2 - 4 tablespoons sweetener*

2 tablespoons tapioca flour

1/2 teaspoon ground black pepper

Zest of 1/2 lemon

Dumplings

1/4 cup coconut flour

3/4 cup almond flour

3 tablespoons cold coconut oil

1 teaspoon baking powder

1/2 teaspoon ground cinnamon

1/4 teaspoon salt

2 eggs

2 tablespoon sweetener

1 teaspoon vanilla

Zest of 1/2 lemon

INSTRUCTIONS

1. For *Dumplings*, sift coconut flour, almond flour, baking powder and salt into small mixing bowl. Cut in cold coconut oil with fork until crumbly. Place in freezer for 10 minutes.

2. Preheat oven to 400 degrees F.

3. For *Blackberry Filling*, add blackberries, sweetener, black pepper and lemon zest to medium pot. Heat over medium heat and bring to simmer. Whisk in tapioca flour and simmer about 10 minutes.

4. Pour hot blackberries into casserole dish and place in hot oven.

5. In medium bowl, beat eggs, sweetener, lemon zest, cinnamon and vanilla. Add chilled flour mixture to eggs and mix until dough comes together.

6. Carefully remove dish from oven and drop 8 dumplings onto bubbling berries.

7. Return dish to oven and bake 15 - 20 min, until dumplings are golden, set and cooked through.

8. Remove dish from oven and allow to cool about 5 minutes.

9. Serve warm. Or allow to cool completely and serve room temperature.

stevia, raw honey or agave nectar

Carrot Cake Cookie Bars

Prep Time: 10 minutes

Cook Time: 25 minutes

Servings: 12

These bars perfectly capture the sweet spiciness of the best carrot cake. Delicious served warm, but you can also wrap them and take them on the go for a satisfying and nourishing snack any time you need a power boost.

INGREDIENTS

2 cups almond meal

2 cups shredded carrots (about 4 large carrots)

3 eggs

1/4 cup coconut oil

1/2 cup unsweetened applesauce

1/2 cup flaked coconut

1/4 cup sweetener*

2 teaspoons vanilla

2 teaspoons ground cinnamon

1 teaspoon ground nutmeg

1/2 teaspoon ground black pepper

1/2 teaspoon salt

INSTRUCTIONS

1. Preheat oven to 350 Degrees F. Line baking pan with parchment or coat lightly with coconut oil.

2. Grate carrots, or process in food processor or bullet blender until finely chopped. Add to medium bowl.

3. Add eggs, oil, applesauce and sweetener to food processor or bullet blender. Process until thickened and light, about 1 - 2 minutes.

4. Pour egg mixture into carrots. Sift in almond flour and salt. Add vanilla and spices. Mix well with a wooden spoon or hand mixer. Stir in coconut.

5. Press dough evenly into prepared baking pan and bake about 25 minutes, or until firm and golden brown.

6. Remove from oven and allow to cool about 10 minutes.

7. Slice into bars and serve warm. Or let cool completely and serve room temperature.

stevia, raw honey, agave nectar or maple syrup

Golden Coconut Cake

Prep Time: 10 minutes

Cook Time: 25 minutes

Servings: 12

This cake will be the guest star of any special occasion—it loves to be the center of attention! It bakes up a to beautiful golden color due to the egg yolks, and the creamy frosting and flaked coconut coating really put it over the top. It will be perfect for your next celebration!

INGREDIENTS

Coconut Cake

6 eggs

3/4 cup coconut flour

1 cup flaked coconut

1 cup unsweetened applesauce

1/2 cup coconut oil

1/2 cup coconut milk

1/2 cup sweetener*

1/2 cup dried pitted dates

2 teaspoons vanilla

1 teaspoon baking soda

1 teaspoon baking powder

1/2 teaspoon salt

Coconut Frosting

1/3 cup coconut cream (from 1 can settled full-fat coconut milk)

2 - 4 tablespoons sweetener*

1/2 teaspoon vanilla

1/2 cup flaked coconut

INSTRUCTIONS

1. Preheat oven to 325°F. Line two or square baking pans with parchment or coat lightly with coconut oil.

2. Add dates, coconut milk, and half of eggs and oil to food processor or bullet blender. Process until dates a broken down, about 1 - 2 minutes.

3. Pour date mixture into medium bowl. Add applesauce, sweetener, vanilla, and remaining eggs and oil. Beat with hand mixer or whisk until well combined.

4. Sift coconut flour, salt, and baking soda and baking powder into wet ingredients. Blend until smooth. Stir in coconut.

5. Pour batter into prepared baking pans and bake for about 25 minutes, or until golden and toothpick inserted into center comes out clean.

6. Remove from oven and allow to cool. Place in refrigerator to speed cooling.

7. For *Coconut Frosting*, beat coconut cream in medium mixing bowl until slightly thickened. Add sweetener and vanilla, and continue to beat until full thickened and fluffy.

8. Frost cooled cakes and stack one on top of the other. Evenly sprinkle flaked coconut on top layer of frosted cake.

9. Slice and serve.

stevia, raw honey, agave nectar or maple syrup

Chocolate Zucchini Cake

Prep Time: 10 minutes

Cook Time: 25 minutes

Servings: 12

This may seem like one of those recipes created to get kids to eat more vegetables by disguising them in sweet treats—but this elegant tea cake stands on its own. Sure, it might get the kids to eat more zucchini but that's not the point. It will also introduce more chocolate into your diet which is definitely a good thing!

INGREDIENTS

1 1/2 cups almond flour

2 eggs

1 medium zucchini (1 1/2 cups grated)

1/2 cup unsweetened applesauce

1/4 cup coconut oil

1/4 - 1/2 cup sweetener*

1/4 cup cocoa powder

2 tablespoons ground chia seed (or flax meal)

1 teaspoon baking soda

1 teaspoon baking powder

1 teaspoon vanilla

1 teaspoon ground cinnamon

1 teaspoon ground black pepper

1/2 teaspoon salt

1/4 cup GF cocoa nibs or chocolate chips (optional)

INSTRUCTIONS

1. Preheat oven to 350 degrees F. Line rectangular baking pan with parchment or lightly coat with coconut oil.

2. Add eggs, coconut oil, applesauce and sweetener to food processor or bullet blender. Process until mixture is thick and lightened.

3. Grate zucchini and add to medium mixing bowl. Pour egg mixture over grated zucchini.

4. Sift almond flour, cocoa powder, chia meal, baking soda and powder, salt and spices into bowl. Beat with hand mixer or whisk to combine. Stir in cocoa nibs or chocolate chips (optional).

5. Pour batter into prepared baking pan and bake for about 25 minutes, until toothpick inserted into center comes out clean.

6. Remove from oven and let cool about 10 minutes.

7. Slice and serve warm. Or let cool completely and serve room temperature.

*stevia, raw honey or agave nectar

Apple Turnover Pastries

Prep Time: 20 minutes

Cook Time: 20 minutes

Servings: 4

These turnovers, fresh from the oven, make an ordinary breakfast or brunch a special event. From the crumbly crust to the tender apple-and-raisin filling this old-fashioned pastry has all the makings of a classic. Make them part of your culinary heritage.

INSTRUCTIONS

Crust

2 cups almond flour

2 eggs

3 tablespoons coconut oil

1 tablespoon sweetener*

1/2 teaspoon baking soda

1/2 teaspoon baking powder

1 teaspoon ground cinnamon

1/4 teaspoon salt

Filling

2 sweet apples

1/4 cup water

1 teaspoon tapioca flour

1 tablespoon ground cinnamon

1/2 teaspoon ground nutmeg

1 teaspoon vanilla

2 tablespoons sweetener * (optional)

2 tablespoons raisins (optional)

2 tablespoons chopped walnuts (optional)

DIRECTIONS

1. For *Crust*, sift almond flour into medium mixing bowl. Add baking soda and powder, cinnamon and salt.

2. Whisk eggs and sweetener in small mixing bowl, then add to flour mixture and combine. Slowly add coconut oil until malleable dough comes together.

3. Roll in plastic wrap or wrap tightly in parchment and refrigerate for 15 minutes.

4. Preheat oven to 400 degrees. Line sheet pan with parchment or baking mat. Cover cutting board with parchment. Heat medium pan over medium-high heat.

5. For *Filling*, peel and dice apples. Add apples to hot pan with water, tapioca, cinnamon, nutmeg, and sweetener and spices (optional).

6. Stir and simmer for about 5 - 8 minutes, until apples are tender and thick glaze forms. Remove from heat and add raisins and chopped walnuts (optional).

7. Remove dough from refrigerator. Roll dough out on parchment covered cutting board to about 1/8 inch thick square with rolling pin. Use sharp knife or pizza cutter to cut dough into 4 squares.

8. Scoop equal portions of *Filling* into center of one side of each dough square. Fold bare half of dough over filled half. Press

edges together and secure seal, letting any trapped air escape. Repeat with remaining dough.

9. Arrange pies on lined sheet pan and bake 15 - 20 minutes, or until dough is golden and cooked through.

10. Serve immediately. Or allow to cool and serve room temperature.

stevia, raw honey or agave nectar

Cocoa Cream Muffins

Prep Time: 10 minutes*

Cook Time: 20 minutes

Servings: 12

If you're feeling nostalgic for those cream-filled chocolate snack cakes of yesteryear, indulge your cravings with this recipe. The rich chocolate cake and the vanilla cream center will bring back the good old days when a chocolate cupcake could solve just about any problem.

INGREDIENTS

1 cup almond flour

1 cup coconut flour

3 eggs

1/2 cup unsweetened applesauce

1/4 cup coconut oil

1/4 cup sweetener*

1 avocado

3 tablespoons cocoa powder

1 tablespoon baking powder

1/4 teaspoon ground black pepper

1 teaspoon salt

Filling

2 cups water

1 cup cashews

3 tablespoons sweetener*

2 tablespoon cocoa powder

2 - 4 tablespoons coconut milk

INSTRUCTIONS

1. *Soak cashews overnight in 2 cups water. Drain and rinse. Set aside.

2. Preheat oven to 350 degrees F. Line muffin pan with paper liners or coat with coconut oil.

3. Slice avocado in half, pit, and scoop flesh into food processor or blender. Add eggs, coconut oil, applesauce and sweetener. Process until smooth.

4. Pour avocado blend into medium mixing bowl. Sift in almond flour, cocoa powder, baking powder, salt and pepper. Beat with hand mixer or whisk until combined.

5. Pour batter into prepared muffin pan. Bake 20 -25 minutes, or until firm but springy in center.

6. For *Filling*, add soaked cashews, sweetener and cocoa powder to food processor or bullet blender. Process until smooth and creamy. Add coconut milk if necessary to reach desired consistency.

7. Remove muffins from oven and let cool.

8. Scoop out center of muffin with knife or teaspoon, and fill with *Filling*. Or transfer *Filling* to pastry bag fitted with 1/2 inch tip, insert tip into muffin and fill.

9. Serve warm or room temperature.

*stevia, raw honey or agave nectar

Ginger Spice Cookies

Prep Time: 15 minutes

Cook Time: 15 minutes

Servings: 6

Picture a stack of these crunchy goodies with a hot cup of tea or cider and you have the essence of autumn. Ginger and spice and everything nice make a satisfying treat any time of the year.

INGREDIENTS

1 1/2 cups almond flour

1 egg

1/4 cup sweetener*

2 tablespoons coconut oil

1 teaspoon ground chia seed (or flax meal)

1/4 teaspoon baking soda

1 tablespoon ground ginger

1/2 teaspoon ground clove

Pinch all spice

Pinch ground black pepper

Pinch salt

INSTRUCTIONS

1. Preheat oven to 350 degrees F. Line sheet pan with parchment or baking mat, or lightly coat with coconut oil.
2. Beat egg, oil, sweetener and chia meal in medium mixing bowl with hand mixer or whisk.

3. Add almond flour, baking soda, salt and spices. Mix until combined.

4. Chill batter in freezer for 5 - 10 minutes.

5. Scoop chilled batter into 6 large rounds on prepared sheet pan. Press into disk shape with hand.

6. Bake for about 15 minutes, until firm around the edges and golden brown.

7. Remove from oven and let cool about 10 minutes.

8. Serve warm. Or let cool completely and serve room temperature.

* raw honey, agave nectar, grade B maple syrup, molasses

Lemon Coconut Bars

Prep Time: 15 minutes

Cook Time: 30 minutes

Servings: 12

Everyone loves lemon bars, and these take them to new heights with the addition of exotic coconut flavors and rich cashews. With a zesty lemon filling and a nutty shortbread crust, these are truly addictive! A nice recipe to serve to guests.

INGREDIENTS

Crust

1/2 cup raw cashews

2/3 cup coconut flour

2 eggs

2 tablespoons coconut oil

2 tablespoons sweetener*

1 tablespoon flaked coconut

1 teaspoon fresh lemon juice

1/2 teaspoon baking soda

1/2 teaspoon vanilla

Filling

2 eggs

2 egg yolks

1 cup fresh lemon juice (about 6 lemons)

1/2 cup sweetener*

1/3 - 1/2 cup flaked coconut

2 tablespoons coconut flour

1 teaspoon lemon zest

INSTRUCTIONS

1. Preheat oven to 350 degrees F. Lightly coat rectangular baking dish with coconut oil, or line with parchment.

2. For *Crust*, add cashews and coconut to food processor or bullet blender and process until finely ground. Add remaining *Crust* ingredients to food processor and pulse until dough comes together.

3. Press dough into bottom of baking dish, and slightly up the sides. Dock crust with fork to prevent bubbling.

4. Place crust in oven and bake for 8 - 10 minutes.

5. For *Filling*, beat eggs, egg yolks, lemon juice, lemon zest and sweetener with hand mixer or whisk in medium bowl.

6. Sift in coconut flour and beat to combine. Let mixture sit for 5 minutes. Add flaked coconut and beat again to combine.

7. Pour *Filling* over par baked crust. Place in oven and bake 20 minutes, until center is set but still slightly jiggly.

8. Remove from oven and let cool for 20 minutes. Refrigerate about 20 minutes, until fully set and chilled.

9. Serve chilled or room temperature.

* raw honey or agave nectar

Sweet Potato Cinnamon Rolls

Prep Time: 10 minutes

Cook Time: 20 minutes

Servings: 8

Possibly the only way to improve on cinnamon rolls is to add mashed sweet potato. The orangey favorite adds a rich tenderness to the dough, and their delicate flavor melds beautifully with the fragrant and sticky cinnamon filling. With a chai latte, you will be transported.

INGREDIENTS

Sweet Potato Roll

1 cup tapioca flour

1/4 - 1/3 cup coconut flour

1 egg

1/2 cup canned yams

1/4 cup warm water

1/4 cup coconut oil

1 - 2 tablespoons sweetener*

1 teaspoon apple cider vinegar

1 teaspoon baking soda

1/2 teaspoon ground cinnamon

1/2 teaspoon nutmeg

1/4 teaspoon ground black pepper

1 teaspoon salt

Cinnamon Swirl

4 - 5 dried pitted dates

1 teaspoon tapioca flour

1 tablespoon ground cinnamon

1/4 cup hot water

INSTRUCTIONS

1. Preheat oven to 350 degrees F. Line muffin pan with paper liners or coat with coconut oil. Heat water in small pan over medium heat. Cover cutting board with parchment.

2. For *Cinnamon Swirl*, add dates, tapioca, cinnamon, and hot water to food processor or bullet blender. Process until dates are broken down and thick mixture forms. Set aside.

3. For *Sweet Potato Roll*, sift tapioca flour, 1/4 cup coconut flour, baking soda, salt and spices into In medium bowl.

4. In small bowl, beat egg, yams, sweetener and vinegar with hand mixer or whisk until well combined. Beat in warm water and oil.

5. Add yam mixture to dry ingredients and mix until well combined. If necessary, add coconut flour or water 1 tablespoon at a time to form a soft and slightly sticky dough.

6. Dust parchment covered cutting board and hands with tapioca flour to prevent sticking. Turn dough out onto parchment. Use dusted hands or rolling pin to flatten dough into 1/2 inch thick square.

7. Use spoon or knife to spread *Cinnamon Swirl* evenly over dough. Roll dough into log and cut into 8 slices, approximately 1 - 1 1/2 inch thick.

8. Turn rolls swirl side up and place in prepared muffin pan.

9. Place in oven and bake about 20 minutes, or until edges browned, cinnamon bubbles, and tops are firm.

10. Remove from oven and let cool about 5 minutes.

11. Serve immediately. Or let cool and serve or room temperature or chilled.

stevia, raw honey or agave nectar

Candied Banana Bread

Prep Time: 5 minutes

Cook Time: 25 minutes

Servings: 9

Delicious bites of caramelized fruit enrich this special baked treat. This is a banana bread unlike any you've had before—this time, it's dressed up and ready to party. This recipe can be made as a loaf—cut it into nice thick slices to really savor the candied bananas!

INGREDIENTS

3/4 cup almond flour

1/2 cup coconut flour

2 eggs

2 overripe bananas

1/4 sweetener*

2 tablespoons coconut oil

1 tablespoons baking powder

1 tablespoon cinnamon

1 teaspoon vanilla

1/2 teaspoon salt

2 firm bananas

4 dried pitted dates

1/4 cup water

INSTRUCTIONS

1. Preheat oven to 350 degrees F. Coat square baking pan with coconut oil or line with parchment.
2. Add pitted dates and water to food processor or bullet blender and process until dates are broken down.
3. Add processed dates to medium pan. Heat pan over medium-high heat.
4. Peel and chop firm bananas. Add to hot dates and sauté until caramelized, about 3 minutes. Remove from heat and set aside.
5. In medium mixing bowl, sift flour, baking powder, cinnamon, vanilla and salt.
6. Beat eggs, overripe bananas, coconut oil and sweetener in separate bowl with hand mixer or whisk. Add to flour mixture and mix to combine. Fold in candied bananas.
7. Pour batter into prepared baking pan and bake for about 25 minutes, or until browned and toothpick inserted into center comes out clean.
8. Let cool at least 5 minutes.
9. Slice and serve warm. Or allow to cool completely and serve room temperature.

NOTE: Bake in oiled loaf pan for about 40 minutes for **Candied Banana Bread** Loaf.

stevia, raw honey or agave nectar

Orange Cranberry Muffins

Prep Time: 5 minutes

Cook Time: 20 minutes

Servings: 12

A little bit sweet, a little bit sour—cranberries and oranges are perfectly piquant. These muffins are lightly sweetened to really bring out the complexity of the fruit. Great for breakfast, but they are elegant enough for an afternoon tea break, too.

INGREDIENTS

1 1/2 cups almond flour

2 eggs

1/2 cup fresh squeezed orange juice (about 2 oranges)

1/4 cup coconut oil

1/4 cup dried cranberries

1 tablespoon orange zest

1 teaspoon baking powder

1/2 teaspoon vanilla

1/2 teaspoon salt

INSTRUCTIONS

1. Preheat oven to 350 degrees F. Line muffin pan with paper liners or coconut oil.
2. In medium bowl, beat eggs with hand mixer or whisk until light and a foamy. Add coconut oil, orange juice and zest. Beat well.

3. Sift in almond flour, baking powder, vanilla and salt. Mix until combined. Stir in cranberries.

4. Use ice cream scoop or tablespoon to scoop batter into prepared muffin pan.

5. Bake about 20 minutes, or until toothpick inserted into center comes out clean.

6. Remove from oven and serve warm. Or let cool completely and serve room temperature.

NOTE: Bake in oiled loaf pan for 40 - 45 minutes for **Cranberry Orange Bread**.

stevia, raw honey or agave nectar

Mocha Brownie Bites

Prep Time: 5 minutes

Cook Time: 25 minutes

Servings: 16

The addition of coffee to this rich brownie batter makes this a more grown-up treat than ordinary brownies. Coffee and chocolate are a classic combination—together they create a subtle, sophisticated flavor that makes them a perfectly "adult" dessert.

INGREDIENTS

4 eggs

1 cup cocoa powder

1/4 cup coconut oil

1/4 cup full-fat coconut milk

1/4 cup sweetener*

2 teaspoons instant espresso (or instant coffee)

1 teaspoon vanilla

INSTRUCTIONS

1. Preheat oven to 350 degrees F. Lightly oil square baking dish or line with parchment.

2. Add eggs, coconut oil, coconut milk and sweetener to medium mixing bowl and beat with hand mixer or whisk. Sift in cocoa powder, espresso and vanilla. Beat until well combined.

3. Pour batter into prepared baking pan and bake for 20 - 25 minutes, until set.

4. Allow to cool completely.

5. Slice and serve room temperature. Or refrigerate and serve chilled.

* raw honey, agave nectar or maple syrup

Blueberry Scones

Prep Time: 5 minutes

Cook Time: 25 minutes

Servings: 8

A true classic. Versatile scones are perfect at breakfast and indispensable at tea time. The addition of blueberries makes them irresistible at any time of day. These are wonderful served warm, and since they come together so quickly, they can be made just before you want to serve them.

INGREDIENTS

2 cups almond flour

1/3 cup arrowroot powder (or tapioca flour)

1 egg

1/2 cup dried or frozen blueberries

1/4 cup coconut oil

2 tablespoons sweetener*

2 teaspoons baking powder

1/2 teaspoon vanilla

1/2 teaspoon salt

1/4 teaspoon ground cinnamon (optional)

INSTRUCTIONS

1. Preheat oven to 350 degrees F. Line sheet pan with parchment or coat with coconut oil.

2. Whisk together almond flour, arrowroot powder, baking powder, salt, vanilla and cinnamon (optional) in medium mixing bowl.

3. In small mixing bowl, beat egg, oil and sweetener with hand mixer or whisk. Add egg mixture to dry ingredients and mix until well combined.

4. Fold in blueberries. Form dough into ball and place on sheet pan . Pat down to flatten to about 1/2 inch thick circle.

5. Cut into eight wedges with pizza cutter or sharp knife. Arrange at least 1 inch apart on sheet pan and bake for 20 - 25 minutes , or until edges are golden brown.

6. Remove from oven and let cool at least 10 minutes.

7. Serve room temperature.

raw honey, agave nectar or grade B maple syrup

Double Pumpkin Muffins

Prep Time: 5 minutes

Cook Time: 25 minutes

Servings: 12

Pumpkins aren't just for jack-o-lanterns! These amazing muffins double the pumpkin by adding nutrient-rich pumpkin seeds! Not only are pumpkin seeds good for you—they are really delicious and add a fun crunch to these tasty treats.

INGREDIENTS

1 3/4 cups coconut flour

2 eggs

15 oz (1 can) pumpkin puree

1 cup unsweetened applesauce

1/2 cup coconut oil

1/4 cup sweetener*

2 teaspoons baking soda

1 1/2 tablespoon ground cinnamon

1/2 teaspoon ground nutmeg

1 teaspoon salt

1/2 cup pumpkin seeds

INSTRUCTIONS

1. Preheat oven to 350 degrees F. Line muffin pan with paper liner or coat with coconut oil.

2. Process eggs, coconut oil, applesauce and sweetener in food processor or blender until thick and light, about 2 minutes.

3. Pour egg mixture into medium mixing bowl. Add pumpkin puree, salt and spices and mix with hand mixer or whisk.

4. Sift in coconut flour and baking soda. Mix until well combined. Stir in half of pumpkin seeds.

5. Pour batter into prepared muffin pan and sprinkle remaining pumpkin seeds over batter.

6. Place in oven and bake 20 - 25 minutes , until edges are golden and tops firm but springy.

7. Remove from oven and allow to cool 5 minutes.

8. Serve warm. Or let cool complete and serve room temperature.

*stevia, raw honey or agave nectar

Cinnamon Raisin Bread

Prep Time: 5 minutes

Cook Time: 20 minutes

Servings: 12

Nothing beats the aroma of fresh-baked cinnamon bread—except the taste! Mix up a loaf or two and enjoy it in all its warm and homey glory.

INGREDIENTS

3/4 cup coconut flour

3/4 cup almond flour

1/4 cup ground chia seed (or flax meal)

2 eggs

1/2 cup raisins

1/2 cup coconut oil

1/2 cup unsweetened applesauce

1/4 cup sweetener*

2 tablespoons ground cinnamon

1 teaspoon baking powder

1 teaspoon salt

1/2 teaspoon ground black pepper (optional)

INSTRUCTIONS

1. Preheat oven to 350 degrees F. Line baking pan with parchment or coat with coconut oil.

2. In large bowl, whisk eggs with hand mixer or whisk until frothy and light. Add coconut oil, sweetener and applesauce. Blend until combined.

3. Sift coconut and almond flour, chia meal, baking powder, salt and spices into wet ingredients. Beat until smooth and well combined. Stir in raisins.

4. Pour batter into prepared baking pan.

5. Bake for 20 - 25 minutes, or until golden brown and firm to the touch.

6. Remove from oven and let cool about 5 minutes.

7. Slice and serve warm. Or allow to cool completely and serve room temperature.

NOTE: Bake in oiled loaf pan for 40 - 45 minutes for **Cinnamon Raison Bread** loaf.

stevia, raw honey or agave nectar

Sandwich Rolls

Prep Time: 5 minutes

Cook Time: 25 minutes

Servings: 4

Every cook needs a good everyday quick bread for sandwiches, and you will quickly add this one to your repertoire. Versatile enough for fillings savory or sweet, these rolls can be used for more than just sandwiches. You will be reaching for this recipe again and again.

INGREDIENTS

Sandwich Rolls

1 cup tapioca flour

1/4 - 1/3 cup coconut flour

1 egg

1/2 cup warm water

1/4 cup coconut oil

1/4 cup unsweetened applesauce

1 teaspoon apple cider vinegar

1/2 teaspoon baking soda

3/4 teaspoon salt

INSTRUCTIONS

1. Preheat oven to 350 degrees F. Line sheet pan with parchment paper or coat with coconut oil. Or coat 4 round mini cake pans with coconut oil.
2. Warm 1/2 cup water in small pot over medium heat.

3. In medium bowl, blend tapioca flour, 1/4 cup coconut flour, baking soda and salt.

4. Add 1 egg, applesauce and coconut oil to food processor or bullet blender. Process about 30 seconds, until a bit light and frothy.

5. Add egg mixture and warm water to flour mixture. Mix until well combined.

6. add coconut flour or water 1 tablespoon at a time to form a soft and slightly sticky dough, if necessary,.

7. Divide dough into 4 portions and roll into round or oblong balls. Dust your hand with extra tapioca flour to prevent sticking.

8. Place rolls on prepared sheet pan and pat down slightly. Brush tops with coconut oil, if preferred.

9. Bake about 25 minutes, or until edges are golden brown and tops are firm.

10. Remove from oven and let cool at least 10 minutes.

11. Slice in half, fill with your favorite cold cuts or hot meats, and serve.

Bagels

Prep Time: 10 minutes

Cook Time: 25 minutes

Servings: 8

You will need a donut pan to bake this other hole-in-the-middle favorite. Although they can't really replace the beloved New York and Montreal versions, these make a handy substitute when an ordinary roll just won't do.

INGREDIENTS

2 cups almond flour

2 tablespoons coconut flour

2 tablespoons ground chia seed (or flax meal)

1 tablespoon tapioca flour (or arrowroot powder)

4 eggs

1/3 cup apple cider vinegar

2 tablespoons unsweetened applesauce

2 tablespoons sweetener*

1 teaspoon baking soda

1/2 teaspoon salt

INSTRUCTIONS

1. Preheat oven to 350 degrees. Lightly coat donut pan with coconut oil.

2. Add almond, coconut and tapioca flours, chia meal, baking soda and salt to food processor or bullet blender, and process for 1 minute.
3. Add eggs, sweetener, applesauce and apple cider vinegar to flour mixture and process until fully blended, about 1 - 2 minutes.
4. Carefully scoop batter into donut pan, avoiding raised middle.
5. Place in oven and bake about 20 - 25 minutes.
6. Remove and let cool about 5 minutes. Then remove from pan.
7. Slice in half and serve immediately. Or let cool completely and serve room temperature.

NOTE: Bake in 8 round mini cake pans lightly coated with coconut oil if you do not have a donut pan.

* stevia, raw honey or agave nectar

All-Purpose Pizza Crust

Prep Time: 5 minutes

Cook Time: 20 minutes

Servings: 2

Pizza is one of the most popular of all dishes because of its versatility, its ease of preparation, and of course, its mixture of flavors and textures. You can top this basic crust with virtually any vegetable or meat, and in a few minutes you will have a savory, crispy meal.

INGREDIENTS

1/3 cup coconut flour

3 eggs

1/2 cup coconut milk

2 tablespoons flax meal (or ground chia seed)

2 tablespoons tapioca flour

1 teaspoon baking powder

1/2 teaspoon salt

INSTRUCTIONS

1. Preheat oven to 350 degrees F. Line sheet pan with parchment paper or baking mat, or coat lightly with coconut oil.
2. In medium bowl, beat eggs and coconut milk with hand mixer or whisk until well combined.
3. Sift coconut and tapioca flour, flax meal, baking powder and salt into egg mixture. Beat into thick batter.
4. Spread batter into desired shape on sheet pan with ladle or spatula.

5. Place in oven and bake for 10 minutes, or until firm enough to flip.

6. Carefully remove par baked crust. Peel away from sheet pan and turn over.

7. Return crust to oven and bake for additional 8 - 10 minutes, or until cooked through.

8. Remove crust and evenly spread with desired sauce and sprinkle with favorite toppings.

9. Set oven to broil. Broil pizza for 1 - 2 minutes, just to heat toppings.

10. Remove pizza and slice with knife or pizza cutter. Serve hot.

Perfectly Pita

Prep Time: 5 minutes

Cook Time: 20 minutes

Servings: 1

Pita bread is an indispensable accompaniment for a number of middle-eastern and European cuisines. These breads are perfect for sandwiches or for dipping. You will want to have plenty on hand for a variety of meals—from mezes to shwarma.

INGREDIENTS

1 cup tapioca flour

1 egg

1/4 cup water

2 tablespoons coconut oil

1 teaspoon ground chia seed (or flax meal)

1/2 teaspoon baking soda

1/4 teaspoon ground white pepper (or black pepper)

1/4 teaspoon salt

INSTRUCTIONS

1. Preheat the oven to 375 degrees F. Line sheet pan with parchment paper or baking mat, or lightly coat with coconut oil. Heat small pot over low heat.

2. Add 1/3 cup tapioca flour, chia meal, water and 1 tablespoon coconut oil to pot. Stir until mixture comes together. Remove from heat and cool in freezer.

3. In medium bowl, blend remaining tapioca flour, baking soda, salt and pepper. Then add egg and remaining oil. Mix until combined.

4. Add cooled chia mixture to bowl. Mix to combine, then remove and knead briefly to bring together dough.

5. Form round disk, then flatten on prepared sheet pan to 1/4 - 1/3 inch with hands or rolling pin.

6. Place in oven and bake about 15 minutes. Carefully remove pan and turn pita over with spatula. Return to oven and bake another 5 - 10 minutes, or until crisp.

7. Remove from oven and fill with favorite Mediterranean meats. Or cut into wedges and dip into favorite spreads.

8. Serve warm or room temperature.

Sesame Pretzel Sticks

Prep Time: 15 minutes

Cook Time: 20 minutes

Servings: 6

Pretzels are an old German beer garden tradition—served with an overflowing mug of something cold and frothy--they are as big as dinner plates. This updated version is decidedly less dramatic, but every bit as tasty. Baking them into sticks make the recipe a snap!

INGREDIENTS

1 cup coconut flour

1/2 cup tapioca flour

1/3 cup coconut oil

2 tablespoons unsweetened applesauce

1/2 cup water

1 egg

2 tablespoons apple cider vinegar

1/2 teaspoon baking soda

1/2 teaspoon baking powder

1/2 teaspoon salt

1 tablespoon sesame seeds

INSTRUCTIONS

1. Preheat oven to 350 degrees F. Heat medium pan over medium-high heat. Line sheet pan with parchment or baking mat.

2. Add coconut oil, water, vinegar and salt to pot. Bring to a boil and remove from heat. Stir in apple sauce.

3. Whisk in tapioca flour. Stir with wooden spoon or soft spatula until mixture gels and comes together.

4. Stir in baking soda and baking powder. Continue mixing for about 1 minute. Mixture will foam and expand. Let mixture sit and cool about 5 minutes.

5. Sift in coconut flour. Mix partially, then beat in egg. Blend until combined. Excess coconut flour may sit in bottom of bowl.

6. Turn out dough onto cutting board dusted with any excess coconut flour from mixture. Knead dough for 2 minutes.

7. Cut dough into 6 equal portions. Roll out pieces into ropes, then lay straight on prepared sheet pan. Use knife to score dough diagonally a few times for presentation.

8. Brush with coconut oil or full-fat coconut milk and sprinkle with sesame seeds.

9. Place sheet pan in oven and bake about 20 - 25 minutes, until cooked through.

10. Serve immediately with favorite dipping sauce. Or allow to cool and serve room temperature.

Breakfast Buns

Prep Time: 15 minutes

Cook Time: 20 minutes

Servings: 4

Bacon and eggs on a bun! You can make these ahead of time and have a great breakfast for those on-the-go days. Puts the drive-thru to shame!

INGREDIENTS

Breakfast Bun

1 cup tapioca flour

1/4 - 1/3 cup coconut flour

1 egg

1/2 cup warm water

1/4 cup coconut oil

Bacon drippings

2 tablespoons applesauce

1 teaspoon apple cider vinegar

1/2 teaspoon baking soda

1/2 teaspoon ground black pepper

1/4 teaspoon salt

Filling

4 eggs

4 slices nitrate-free bacon

1/2 small bell pepper

1/2 small onion

1/4 teaspoon ground black pepper

1/4 teaspoon salt

INSTRUCTIONS

1. Preheat oven to 350 degrees F. Line sheet pan with parchment paper or coat with coconut oil. Heat medium skillet over medium-high heat. Add water to small pot and heat over medium heat.

2. For *Filling*, peel onion, stem, seed and vein pepper, and chop bacon. Add bacon to hot skillet and sauté until bacon is crisp and almost cooked through. Drain off drippings and set aside.

3. Dice onion and pepper and add to bacon. Sauté about 2 minutes, unto bacon is cooked through and veggies are softened. Add eggs and lightly scrambled, just 30 seconds - 1 minute. Remove from heat and set aside.

4. For *Breakfast Bun*, sift together tapioca flour, coconut flour, baking soda, salt and pepper in medium bowl.

5. Whisk egg, applesauce and vinegar in small bowl. Whisk in warm water, coconut oil and bacon drippings.

6. Add egg mixture to flour mixture and mix until well combined. Add 1 tablespoon coconut flour or water at a time if needed to form soft and slightly sticky dough.

7. Divide dough into 4 portions and flatten into round disks. Dust your hand or rolling pin with extra tapioca flour to prevent sticking.

8. Scoop loose egg *Filling* into center of each dough disk and pinch edges of dough together to create round, sealed ball.

9. Place filled buns sealed side down on sheet pan and pat down slightly.

10. Place in oven and bake 20 minutes, or until edges are golden brown and dough is cooked through.

11. Remove from oven and let cool about 5 minutes.

12. Serve warm.

Avocado Club Muffin

Prep Time: 10 minutes

Cook Time: 15 minutes

Servings: 12

This bread is unusual and versatile! Serve with eggs for a delicious brunch, or bake into a loaf. Sliced thin, it makes a great base for all sorts of savory toppings and is perfect for entertaining as it can be used to make excellent hors d'oeuvres.

INGREDIENTS

1 cup almond flour

2 eggs

1 avocado

4 slices nitrate-free bacon

1 tablespoon sweetener*

1 teaspoon apple cider vinegar

1 teaspoon baking powder

1/4 teaspoon ground white pepper (or black pepper)

INSTRUCTIONS

1. Preheat oven to 350 degrees F. Line muffin pan with paper liners or light coat with coconut oil. Heat medium pan over medium-high heat.

2. Finely chop bacon and add to hot pan. Sauté until crisp and cooked through, about 5 minutes. Set aside.

3. Beat eggs, sweetener and vinegar in medium mixing bowl with hand mixer or whisk until thick and slightly foamy.

4. Slice avocado in half. Scoop flesh of one half into egg mixture. Add bacon and drippings, almond flour, baking powder and black pepper and mix until combined.

5. Dice remaining avocado flesh and fold into batter.

6. Use ice cream scoop or tablespoon to scoop batter into prepared muffin pan.

7. Bake about 15 - 20 minutes, until edges are golden brown and tops are firm.

8. Remove from oven and let cool for 5 minutes.

9. Serve warm. Or cool completely and serve temperature.

NOTE: Bake in square oiled baking pan for 30 - 35 minutes for **Avocado Club Bread**.

stevia, raw honey or agave nectar

Chicken Dumpling Bun

Prep Time: 15 minutes

Cook Time: 20 minutes

Servings: 4

With a delicious chicken filling, these buns make a great light meal or snack. Chicken and dumplings is a long-time favorite for good reason—and this recipe captures the flavors of chicken and vegetables that are so well loved.

INGREDIENTS

Dumpling Bun

1 cup tapioca flour

1/4 - 1/3 cup coconut flour

1 egg

1/2 cup warm GF chicken stock

1/4 cup coconut oil

1/4 cup applesauce

1 teaspoon apple cider vinegar

1 teaspoon baking soda

1/2 teaspoon onion powder

1/ 4 teaspoon garlic powder

1/2 teaspoon salt

Filling

8 oz boneless chicken (breasts, thighs, etc.)

1 small carrot

1 small celery stalk

1/2 teaspoon dried thyme

1/4 teaspoon ground sage

1/2 teaspoon ground black pepper

1/2 teaspoon salt

INSTRUCTIONS

1. Preheat oven to 350 degrees F. Line sheet pan with parchment paper or coat with coconut oil. Heat medium skillet over medium heat and lightly coat with coconut oil.

2. Add chicken stock to small pot and heat over medium heat.

3. For *Filling*, dice carrot and celery, fillet chicken in half, and add to hot oiled skillet with salt and spices. Sauté until chicken is cooked through and browned and veggies are softened, about 5 - 8 minutes. Remove from heat and set aside. Shred or dice rested chicken and mix thoroughly with sautéed veggies.

4. For *Dumpling Bun*, sift together tapioca flour, coconut flour, baking soda, salt and spices in medium bowl.

5. Whisk egg, applesauce and vinegar in small bowl. Whisk in warm chicken stock and coconut oil.

6. Add egg mixture to flour mixture and mix until well combined. Add 1 tablespoon coconut flour or water at a time if needed to form soft and slightly sticky dough.

7. Divide dough into 4 portions and flatten into round disks. Dust your hand or rolling pin with extra tapioca flour to prevent sticking.

8. Scoop chicken *Filling* into center of each dough disk and pinch edges of dough together to create round, sealed ball.

9. Place filled buns sealed side down on sheet pan and pat down slightly.

10. Place in oven and bake 20 minutes, or until edges are golden brown and dough is cooked through.

11. Remove from oven and let cool about 5 minutes.

12. Serve warm.

Lemon Poppy Seed Muffins

Prep Time: 5 minutes

Cook Time: 20 minutes

Servings: 12

What a delightful combination! Ancient peoples used poppy seeds to flavor food and for medicinal purposes, and poppy seeds are often used in cuisines of eastern Europe where they are prized for their flavor and color. Lemons and poppy seeds naturally bring out the best in each other and these muffins will convince you they belong together.

INGREDIENTS

6 eggs

1/2 cup coconut flour

1/4 cup coconut oil

1/4 cup sweetener*

1 teaspoon vanilla

1 teaspoon poppy seeds

1/2 teaspoon baking soda

Juice of 2 lemons

Zest of 2 lemons

INSTRUCTIONS

1. Preheat oven to 350 degrees F. Oil muffin pan or line with paper liners.

2. Zest, *then* juice 2 lemons. Add to large mixing bowl with eggs, coconut oil, sweetener and vanilla. Beat with hand mixer or whisk until well combined.

3. Sift coconut flour and baking soda into wet ingredients, and mix until smooth. Stir in poppy seeds.

4. Use ice cream scoop or tablespoon to pour batter into prepared muffin pan.

5. Place in oven and bake for about 20 minutes, or until golden around edges and toothpick inserted into middle comes out clean.

6. Remove from oven and let cool for 5 minutes.

7. Serve warm. Or allow to cool completely and serve room temperature.

* raw honey or agave nectar

Gluten Free Desserts

Flourless Chocolate Cake

Prep Time: 15 minutes

Cook Time: 30 minutes

Servings: 8

It sometimes seems that flourless chocolate cake was invented to keep us GFs from sinking into a pool of dark despair—by giving us a chance to sink into a pool of dark decadence instead! Actually, the idea has been around long time—well before we were hungering for desserts that were every bit as sinfully delicious as those we had to give up. This achingly rich, meltingly smooth delight is completely free of wheat—something a lot of other so-called flourless chocolate cakes can't really claim. Indulge in a piece soon, perhaps garnished with some raspberries and savor how satisfying living GF can be

INGREDIENTS

16 oz organic bittersweet chocolate

1/4 cup cocoa powder

6 eggs

1 cup coconut or other cooking oil

3/4 cup sweetener*

2 tablespoons water

2 teaspoons vanilla

1/4 teaspoon salt

INSTRUCTIONS

1. Preheat oven to 275 degrees F. Coat 2 mini springform pans with oil, then dust with cocoa powder, and cover the outside base of the pans with aluminum foil. Or line muffin pan with

paper liners, or leave bare and coat liners or bare pan with oil and dust with cocoa powder.

2. Slowly melt chocolate and oil over a double boiler, heated over medium heat. Do not boil water in bottom of double boiler. Stir frequently.

3. Remove from heat once chocolate is melted and beat in sweetener, water, vanilla, salt and any remaining cocoa powder with hand mixer or whisk.

4. Beat in eggs one at a time until thoroughly incorporated.

5. Pour batter into vessels and bake for about 25 - 30 minutes, until set. Cakes will still appear a bit glossy and wet in the middle.

6. Cool for 30 minutes, then refrigerate at least 2 hours before serving.

7. Cut springform cakes with a knife warmed until hot running water, then dried.

8. Serve chilled or room temperature.

maple syrup, raw honey or agave nectar. Granulated sugar can be used instead. See note for tips on substituting dry sweetener for liquid.

Apple Dump Muffins

Prep Time: 15 minutes

Cook Time: 25 minutes

Servings: 12

I know what you're thinking: Something with the word "dump" in the title sounds very suspicious! But dump muffins and cakes are perfectly scrumptious, and a time-honored tradition of the pressed-for-time cook. Those very busy mothers of the past did not want fussy recipes and fiddly techniques--forget about separating egg whites and creaming butter and sugar. Grab a bowl, dump in the ingredients, give it a quick stir, scrape it into a baking pan, and put it on the fire. So easy, you could even do it while blazing a Westward trail.

INGREDIENTS

6 medium apples, peeled, cored, and thinly sliced

1 cup almond flour

1/4 cup tapioca flour

3 eggs

1/2 cup coconut or other cooking oil

1/2 cup sweetener*

2 teaspoons baking powder

2 tablespoons ground cinnamon

1 teaspoon ground nutmeg

1 teaspoon salt

1/2 teaspoon black pepper (or white pepper)

Juice of one-half lemon

INSTRUCTIONS

1. Preheat oven to 350 degrees F. Lightly coat muffin pan with oil, or line with paper liners.

2. Peel, core and thinly slice apples. Add to medium bowl with 1 tablespoon cinnamon and juice of half a lemon. Evenly sprinkle on tapioca flour and carefully toss with hands to coat apples.

3. In medium mixing bowl, blend almond flour, baking powder, spices and salt. Beat in eggs, sweetener and oil with hand mixer or whisk. Fold in sliced apples.

4. Scoop batter into muffin pan and bake for 20 -25 minutes, or until top is browned and firm but springy. A toothpick inserted into the center should come our moist but clean.

5. Serve warm solo, or drizzled with your favorite sweetener.

NOTE: For *Apple Dump Cake*, bake in square baking dish or Bundt pan for 40 - 50 minutes.

maple syrup, raw honey or agave nectar. Granulated sugar can be used instead. See note for tips on substituting dry sweetener for liquid.

Pumpkin Spice Cakes

Prep Time: 5 minutes

Cook Time: 15 minutes

Servings: 12

Not just for pies and jack-o-lanterns, the squash family's most exuberant performer also gives us these autumnal delights. Sugar and spice, and a whole lot of beta-carotene, these muffins are moist, yummy, and have the added crunch and nuttiness of pumpkin seeds! Double the pumpkin punch.

INGREDIENTS

3/4 cup coconut flour

4 eggs

1/4 cup coconut or other cooking oil

1/2 cup sweetener*

1/2 cup pumpkin purée

1 teaspoon baking soda

1 tablespoon ground cinnamon

1 tablespoon ground ginger

1 tablespoon ground nutmeg

1 tablespoon ground black pepper

1 teaspoon vanilla

1/2 teaspoon salt

1/4 cup roasted pumpkin seeds

INSTRUCTIONS

1. Preheat oven to 350 degrees F. Lightly coat 4 mini cake pans or mini loaf pans with oil, or line with parchment paper.
2. Sift coconut flour, baking soda, salt and spices into large mixing bowl.
3. In medium mixing bowl, beat egg whites to soft peaks with hand mixer or whisk. About 5 minutes.
4. Then beat in yolks, oil, sweetener and pumpkin purée. Mix wet ingredients into dry blend until combined.
5. Pour batter into mini cake loaf pans and sprinkle on pumpkin seeds.
6. Bake for 20 - 25 minutes, or until firm but springy in the center and browned. A toothpick inserted into the middle should come out clean.
7. Remove from oven and allow to cool for 5 minutes before serving.
8. Serve warm or room temperature.

NOTE: For large **Pumpkin Spice Cake**, oil large loaf pan or springform pan and bake 40 - 45 minutes.

maple syrup, raw honey or agave nectar. Granulated sugar can be used instead. See note for tips on substituting dry sweetener for liquid.

Fruit And Nut Cake

Prep Time: 10 minutes

Cook Time: 25 minutes

Servings: 8

Forget about those mail-order bricks of Yuletides past. More like the punch-line to a joke about a "gag" gift than a genuine token of esteem, those gummy, artificially-flavored, and garishly-colored little bakeshop horrors earned their bad reputation. After you taste this exquisite gem-like treat, however, you will understand why Fruit and Nut Cake became a holiday favorite in the first place. Replacing the wheat flour with almond flour really brings out the concentrated winey flavors of the dried cherries and other fruits. Now who's laughing at fruit cake?

INGREDIENTS

1 1/2 cup almond flour

4 eggs

2 tablespoons coconut or other cooking oil

Juice of orange half

1/4 cup sweetener*

1/2 cup walnuts

1/4 cup pecans

1/2 cup dried pitted dates

1/2 cup dried cherries

1/4 cup dried apricots

1/4 cup raisins

1/2 teaspoon baking soda

1 teaspoon ground ginger

1 teaspoon vanilla

1/2 teaspoon salt

Zest of orange half

INSTRUCTIONS

1. Preheat oven to 350 degrees F. Lightly coat 2 small loaf pans or one Bundt pan with oil.

2. Sift almond flour, baking soda and salt into large mixing bowl.

3. Chop walnuts, pecans, apricots and dates. Then stir all dried fruit and nuts into flour mixture.

4. In medium mixing bowl, mix eggs, oil, juice and zest of half an orange, sweetener, ginger and vanilla. Then pour and mix into dry ingredients until just combined.

5. Scoop batter into loaf pans or Bundt pan, and smooth tops with spatula.

6. Bake 20 - 30 minutes, or until firm, browned and firm in the center.

7. Remove from oven and allow to cool before slicing.

8. Serve warm or room temperature.

stevia, maple syrup, raw honey or agave nectar. Granulated sugar or stevia can be used instead. See note for tips on substituting dry sweetener for liquid.

Toasted Almond Cream Cakes

Prep Time: 15 minutes*

Cook Time: 20 minutes

Servings: 12

These light and airy cakes will remind you of the French teatime favorites, *financiers*. Imagine enjoying these almond *frangipane*-cream-filled delights while sipping a lovely tisane in Paris. Make them your own version of the evocative *madeleine,* and be transported.

INGREDIENTS

Cake

1 cup almond flour

4 egg whites

1/3 cup coconut or other cooking oil

1/4 cup almond milk

1/4 cup sweetener*

1 teaspoon baking powder

1/4 cup slice almonds

Almond Cream

2 cups skinless almonds

1/4 cup sweetener

1 teaspoon vanilla

Water

INSTRUCTIONS

1. *Soak almonds overnight in water. Drain and rinse.

2. Preheat the oven to 350 degrees F. Heat medium pan over medium heat. Lightly coat muffin pan with oil, or line with paper liners

3. Add almond flour to hot dry pan and toast about 5 minutes, stirring frequently. Do not burn. Remove from heat and set aside.

4. Beat egg whites to soft peaks with hand mixer or whisk in medium bowl. Then beat in oil, milk and 1/4 cup sweetener. Sift in toasted almond flour and baking powder. Mix until just combined.

5. Use ice cream scoop or spoon to scoop batter into muffin pan. Each cup should be only 1/2 full.

6. Bake about 15 minutes, or until center is set but springy.

7. Remove pan from oven and remove cakes from pan. Let cool for about 15 minutes.

8. While cakes cool, blend soaked almonds, 1/4 cup sweetener, 1 teaspoon vanilla and water as needed in food processor or blender to make smooth *Almond Cream*.

9. Wipe out pan with paper towel and return dry pan to medium heat. Toast slice almonds about 5 minutes, until aromatic and golden. Do not burn. Remove from heat and set aside.

10. When cakes are cooled, slice in half to create top and bottom layer. Scoop cream onto bottom half, and top with top half of cake. Scoop another dollop of cream over top half and sprinkle on slice toasted almonds.

11. Serve room temperature.

NOTE: For large **Toasted Almond Cream Cake** , bake batter in 2 round cake pans for 35 - 40 minutes.

maple syrup, raw honey or agave nectar. Granulated sugar can be used instead. See note for tips on substituting dry sweetener for liquid.

Pineapple Upside Down Cake

Prep Time: 15 minutes

Cook Time: 30 minutes

Servings: 12

Get your Gatsby on with this classic dessert! The "roaring 1920s" ushered in all sorts of new products from far-off lands, with exotic and sweet pineapple being all the rage. The first printed recipe for Pineapple Upside Down Cake appeared in 1924, and it combined the modern wonder of factory-sliced and canned pineapple with good old-fashioned skillet cake—all in a glorious Art Deco design. With a bright red Maraschino cherry on top, it was a hugely popular emblem of the modernity the era is famed for—and it has remained a homey and deliciously gooey favorite ever since.

INGREDIENTS

2 cups almond flour

8 - 12 slices canned pineapple in juice

8 - 12 pitted cherries

1/4 cup sweetener*

3 eggs

1/4 cup coconut or other cooking oil

1/2 cup pineapple juice (reserved from can)

2 teaspoons baking soda

2 teaspoons vanilla

1/2 teaspoon salt

INSTRUCTIONS

1. Preheat oven to 350 degrees F. Line 9x13 baking dish with parchment paper, or coat with coconut oil.

2. Arrange pineapple slices and cherries on bottom of baking dish. Place in oven while you prepare the batter.

3. Beat egg whites to stiff peaks with hand mixer or whisk in medium mixing bowl. About 7 - 10 minutes.

4. In large mixing bowl, mix yolks, oil, sweetener, pineapple juice and vanilla.

5. Sift almond flour, baking soda and salt into yolk mixture. Beat until well combined.

6. Fold egg whites into batter until evenly combined.

7. Remove hot baking pan from oven, and spread light batter over pineapple and cherries. Smooth top with spatula.

8. Bake for 25 - 30 minutes, or until cake golden brown and firm but springy in the center. A toothpick inserted into the center should come out clean.

9. Remove pan from oven and allow to cool for 15 minutes. Turn cake out onto serving dish and remove parchment. Or scrape any stuck fruit from the pan and place back on cake.

10. Allow to cool another 15 minutes before serving. Serve room temperature or warm.

NOTE: For **Pineapple Upside Dow Cupcakes** , add a pineapple slice and cherry to muffin pan lined with paper liners or coated with oil, then fill cups 2/3 full with batter and bake about 20 minutes.

*stevia, maple syrup, raw honey or agave nectar. Granulated sugar or stevia can be used instead. See note for tips on substituting dry sweetener for liquid.

Banana Bread Pudding

Prep Time: 10 minutes

Cook Time: 30 minutes

Servings: 12

Bread pudding—a rather ingenious way of transforming odd bits of the old-and-stale into a lush and comforting treat is made new here with banana-flavored custard and banana muffins. Frugal cooks have always known that banana bread was an excellent way to salvage over-ripe fruit before it shriveled up and faded away completely. This delicious dish truly makes a virtue of necessity as it elevates repurposing, re-using, and re-cycling into culinary artistry in this fragrant baked custard.

INGREDIENTS

Banana Bread

1 cup of almond flour

2 eggs

2 overripe bananas

1/4 cup sweetener*

2 tablespoons coconut or other cooking oil

1 tablespoon baking powder

1 tablespoon cinnamon

1 teaspoon nutmeg

1 teaspoon vanilla

1/2 teaspoon of salt

Banana Custard

13 oz (1 can) full-fat coconut milk

6 egg yolks

1 overripe banana

1/4 cup sweetener*

1/4 cup raisins

1/2 cup dried pitted dates

2 tablespoons tapioca starch/flour

2 teaspoons vanilla

1 teaspoon cinnamon

Pinch salt

INSTRUCTIONS

1. Preheat oven to 350 degrees F. Line muffin pan with paper liners or coat with oil.
2. In medium mixing bowl, beat 2 eggs, 2 bananas, 2 tablespoons oil and 1/4 cup sweetener with hand mixer or whisk.
3. In separate mixing bowl, add 1 cup almond flour, 1 tablespoon baking powder,1 tablespoon cinnamon, 1 teaspoon nutmeg, 1 teaspoon vanilla and 1/2 teaspoon salt.
4. Pour banana mixture into flour mixture and mix well.
5. Pour batter into muffin pan and bake for about 15 minutes, or until golden brown, risen and firm.
6. While muffins cook, add coconut milk, egg yolks, banana, sweetener, vanilla, cinnamon and salt to medium bowl and blend briefly with hand mixer or whisk.
7. Pour into medium pot and heat over medium heat. Chop dates and add to pot with raisins.

8. Stir in tapioca flour. Stir as *Banana Custard* thickens, about 5 minutes. Remove from heat.

9. Remove muffins from oven and turn out onto cutting board.

10. Increase oven to 375 degrees F. Lightly coat square or rectangular baking dish with oil.

11. Carefully remove paper liners and roughly chop muffins. Add muffin chunks to baking dish. Pour banana custard over chopped muffins.

12. Place dish in oven and bake for 15 minutes.

13. Remove and allow to cool for 15 minutes before serving.

14. Serve warm or room temperature.

stevia, maple syrup, raw honey or agave nectar. Granulated sugar or stevia can be used instead. See note for tips on substituting dry sweetener for liquid.

Simply Sweet Potato Blondie

Prep Time: 15 minutes

Cook Time: 30 minutes

Servings: 12

You just will not believe how luscious this unlikely combo of sweet potato, cacao butter, and coconut are as they come together to create both an homage to the classic brown-sugar based bar cookie, and at the same time turn, it into something far more complex, seductive, and fresh. Try sprinkling the top with a bit of sea salt. You will have to hide these.

INGREDIENTS

2/3 cups coconut flour

2 tablespoons arrowroot powder

1 large sweet potato

4 eggs

3/4 cup sweetener*

1/4 cup full-fat coconut milk

1/4 cup cacao butter

1/2 teaspoon baking powder

2 tablespoons vanilla

Pinch salt

Pinch ground white pepper (or black pepper)

INSTRUCTIONS

1. Preheat oven to 350 degrees F. Grease an 9 x 13 inch pan or "all-corner" specialty brownie pan with oil. Bring medium pot of lightly salted water to boil.

2. Peel and dice sweet potato. Add to boiling water for 5 - 10 minutes, until soft.

3. Beat eggs in medium mixing bowl with hand mixer or whisk. Add sweetener, coconut milk, vanilla and pepper until combined.

4. Sift in flour, arrowroot powder, baking powder and salt, and mix until combined.

5. Drain sweet potatoes and add to small mixing bowl with cacao butter. Beat or mash until cacao butter is well melted. Add sweet potato mixture to egg mixture.

6. Scrape batter into baking pan and smooth top with spatula.

7. Bake for 25 - 30 minutes, until center is firm and top is golden brown. Toothpick inserted into center will come out moist but mostly clean.

8. Allow to cool about 10 minutes. Slice and serve warm or room temperature.

stevia, maple syrup, raw honey or agave nectar. Granulated sugar or stevia can be used instead. See note for tips on substituting dry sweetener for liquid.

Coconut Cream Pie

Prep Time: 20 minutes*

Cook Time: 20 minutes

Servings: 8

A crunchy nut crust lends this old stand-by a trendy new sheen. Coconut and almonds bring out the best in each other—something that a beloved candy bar already demonstrated many years ago. Sometimes you feel like a nut, and sometimes you feel like a Coconut Cream Pie with an almond crust. Drizzle the top with a bit of melted bittersweet chocolate if you're feeling bold.

INGREDIENTS

Crust

1/2 cup soft nuts**

1 cup almond flour

2 teaspoons sweetener***

1/4 - 1/2 cup coconut or other cooking oil

Filling

26 oz (2 cans) full-fat coconut milk

2 eggs

1/2 cup arrowroot powder

1/4 cup sweetener*

1 tablespoon vanilla

1 cup flaked coconut

Pinch salt

INSTRUCTIONS

1. Preheat oven to 350 degrees F. Lightly coast pie plate with oil.

2. Grind nuts into coarse meal with food processor or bullet blender. Add to small bowl with almond flour, 2 tablespoons sweetener and enough oil to bring together soft but crumbly dough.

3. Press dough into pie plate and bake about 10 - 15 minutes, until crust becomes golden.

4. Remove crust from oven and allow to cool. Turn off oven.

5. Add coconut milk, eggs, arrowroot powder, sweetener, vanilla and salt to medium pot. Heat pot over medium heat and bring to a boil. Stir constantly as mixture thickens.

6. Stir in 1/2 cup shredded coconut. Then pour the filling over the crust.

7. *Refrigerate pie until filling is set, about 4 hours.

8. Heat medium pan over medium heat. Add 1/2 cup flaked coconut and toast about 5 minutes. Stir frequently to prevent burning.

9. Sprinkle toasted coconut over pie and serve chilled.

NOTE: Line springform pan with parchment and bake crust, then fill with coconut cream filling for another version of **Coconut Cream Pie**.

*coconut flakes, pecans, walnuts, cashews or brazil nuts
***stevia, maple syrup, raw honey or agave nectar. Granulated sugar or stevia can be used instead. See note for tips on substituting dry sweetener for liquid.

Pecan Chess Pies

Prep Time: 20 minutes

Cook Time: 25 minutes

Servings: 6

Not chess pieces—chess pie! This traditional pastry has nothing to do with "chess," the slightly nerdy, slightly cool, board game. Chess Pies go way back to the Colonial days when people kept their precious desserts tucked away in a safe, or a chest— which is probably how it got its odd name. The Chess Pie is related to the equally-venerable vinegar pie and the Southern favorite, pecan pie, but the addition of coconut milk (or buttermilk, more traditionally) is what gives it its distinctive flavor. Pecans aren't typical of Chess Pie, but they certainly add a buttery richness and help mellow the frank sweetness of the pie. Thankfully, there is no vinegar involved here.

INGREDIENTS

Crust

1 1/2 cups almond flour

1/2 cup pecans

1 egg

2 tablespoons coconut or other oil

1/4 teaspoon salt

Filling

1 cup full-fat coconut milk

2 cups pecans

1 cup dried pitted dates

1/2 cup sweetener*

2 eggs

2 egg yolks

1 1/2 tablespoons arrowroot powder

2 tablespoons coconut or other cooking oil

1 teaspoon vanilla

INSTRUCTIONS

1. Preheat oven to 350 degrees F. Coat 6 mini pie plates or pie pans with oil. Bring small pot of water to boil, leaving room for dates.

2. Add dates to boiling water for about 5 - 10 minutes, until tender. Then drain.

3. For *Crust*, process pecans in food processor or bullet lender until well ground. Add to small mixing bowl with almond flour and salt. Mix in oil and egg until dough forms.

4. Press dough into pie plates with hand or wooden spoon. Bake about 10 minutes, until golden. Remove pie shells from oven and set aside.

5. Chop 1 cup pecans and set aside

6. For *Filling*, process softened dates in food processor or bullet blender with about half of coconut milk. Add to medium mixing bowl with remaining coconut milk, sweetener, eggs, egg yolks, oil, vanilla and arrowroot powder. Beat with hand mixer or whisk until combined and a bit airy. Mix in chopped pecans.

7. Pour batter into mini pie crusts. Top with whole pecans and bake for 20 - 25 minutes, until filling is set.

8. Remove pies and let cool about 20 minutes before serving.

9. Serve warm. Or refrigerate and serve cold. Also great at room temperature.

stevia, raw honey or agave nectar. Granulated sugar or stevia can be used instead. See note for tips on substituting dry sweetener for liquid.

NOTE: For large **Pecan Chess Pie**, bake in 9-inch pie plate for 45 - 55 minutes, or until center is set.

Wild Mince Meat Pie

Prep Time: 20 minutes

Cook Time: 30 minutes

Servings: 8

Although they've never really gained a following in the U.S., in other parts of the anglophone world , mince pies are eagerly awaited each fall. A beloved holiday treat, they have their roots in the medieval period when spices were beginning to shake the European world out of its bland and boring culinary routine. The Puritans banned these sinful and indulgent sweet/ savory treats on religious grounds, and poor penitent wheat-avoiders have had to live under that old prohibition for too long. Until now. Let the idolatry begin.

INGREDIENTS

Crust

4 cups almond flour

2 eggs

1/4 cup coconut or other oil

1/2 teaspoon Celtic sea salt

Filling

12 oz grass-fed beef

2 sweet apples

2 tart apples

1 cup GF beef stock

1/4 cup sweetener*

Juice of 1 orange

Zest of 1 orange

1/4 cup arrowroot powder

1/4 cup apple cider vinegar

1 cup raisins

1/2 cup dried pitted dates

1/2 cup dried pitted prunes

1/2 cup dried cherries

2 teaspoons ground cinnamon

1 teaspoon ground nutmeg

1/2 teaspoon ground cloves

1/2 teaspoon ground black pepper

1/2 teaspoon salt

INSTRUCTIONS

1. Preheat oven to 350 degrees F. Heat large pot over medium-high heat and lightly coat with oil. Lightly oil pie plate. Prepare 4 sheets of parchment.

2. Place beef in hot oiled pan and brown on each side for about 5 - 7 minutes, until just cooked through. Remove beef and set aside. Add beef stock to pot.

3. Mix all *Crust* ingredients together in medium bowl until dough forms. Divide dough in half and use rolling pin to roll dough between two parchment sheets into circles to fit about 1 inch over pie plate.

4. Press one dough circle into pie plate. Crimp edges to create small lip. Bake for 5 minutes, then remove and set aside.

5. Peel, core and grate or dice apples. Add to beef stock with sweetener, zest and juice of orange, vinegar, raisins, cherries, spices and salt. Dice beef, prunes and dates, and add to pot. Stir in arrowroot powder and thicken for a few minutes.

6. Once mixture comes together pour into par-baked pie shell. Top with second dough sheet and crimp edges to fit into bottom crust.

7. Use sharp knife to slice top crust a few times for venting.

8. Bake pie for 30 minutes, or until crust is golden brown.

9. Remove from oven and allow to cool for about 20 minutes.

10. Slice and serve warm. Or allow to cool completely and serve room temperature.

*stevia, raw honey or agave nectar. Granulated sugar or stevia can be used instead. See note for tips on substituting dry sweetener for liquid.

Almond Butter Balls

Prep Time: 10 minutes

Cook Time: 10 minutes

Servings: 12

Closer to a truffle than a cookie, these make spectacular additions to your holiday dessert tray. Try placing them in mini cupcake liners and packaging them into small cardboard boxes for a thoughtful and yummy homemade gift.

INGREDIENTS

1/2 cup almond butter

1/2 cup almonds

1/4 cup cashews

1 tablespoon cocoa powder

1 tablespoon ground chia seed (or flax meal)

5 dried pitted dates

3/4 cup flaked coconut

2 tablespoons sweetener*

1 teaspoon cinnamon

INSTRUCTIONS

1. Heat small pot over high heat. Add cashews and enough water to cover. Boil cashews until softened, about 8 minutes.

2. Add softened cashews to food processor or bullet blender with sweetener, and process until smooth. Add water to thin if mixture is too thick or chunky. Scrape into small mixing bowl.

3. Chop dates and almonds by hand or in food processor or bullet blender. Add to cashew cream with almond butter and mix together.
4. Add cocoa powder, chia or flax meal, coconut and cinnamon, and blend.
5. Add 1 tablespoon at a time of almond butter or cocoa powder to get mixture to perfect consistency to hold together as a ball.
6. Use mini scoop or tablespoon to portion twelve servings. Roll each serving into a ball. Place balls on parchment covered half sheet pan or plate and refrigerate for about 20 minutes.
7. Serve chilled or room temperature.

*stevia, raw honey or agave nectar. Granulated sugar or stevia can be used instead. See note for tips on substituting dry sweetener for liquid.

Spiced Baked Peaches

Prep Time: 5 minutes

Cook Time: 25 minutes

Servings: 4

A brilliant use for less-than-perfect peaches. With a little heat, and a little care, they will simply ooze a spicy and sweet perfume. Good any time of day from breakfast to dinner. And, if you do have perfect fruit, then feel free to gild the lily and heartily enjoy this recipe made with summer's bounty.

INGREDIENTS

2 ripe peaches

1/4 cup walnuts

1/4 cup dried cranberries

2 tablespoons sweetener*

Juice of 1 orange

Zest of 1 orange

1 teaspoon cinnamon

1/2 teaspoon nutmeg

1/2 teaspoon ground allspice

INSTRUCTIONS

1. Preheat oven to 375 degrees F.
2. Slice peaches in half and remove pit. Place peach halves into glass or ceramic baking dish just big enough for them to fit snugly.

3. Chop walnuts and toss with cranberries, sweetener, spices, juice and zest of orange in small bowl.
4. Fill peach halves with fruit and nut mixture. Pour excess liquid over peaches.
5. Bake in oven for about 20 - 25 minutes, until peaches are soften and lightly browned.
6. Remove from oven and let cool about 5 minutes.
7. Serve warm or room temperature.

*stevia, raw honey or agave nectar. Granulated sugar or stevia can be used instead. See note for tips on substituting dry sweetener for liquid.

Perfectly Nutty Refrigerator Fudge

Prep Time: 10* minutes

Cook Time: 5 minutes

Servings: 6

Old fashioned nutty fudge—the kind that you remember from state fairs and family reunions. This recipe is free of all the junky stuff like marshmallow crème that made it an unwelcome intruder at the healthy table, and instead depends on almond and hazelnut butters for its dense and unctuously smooth texture. Not cloyingly sweet—just a satisfying trip down memory lane.

INGREDIENTS

1/4 cup cocoa powder

1/2 cup almond butter (or 3/4 cup almonds)

1/2 cup hazelnut butter (or 1/2 cup hazelnuts)

2 tablespoons coconut or other cooking oil

1/4 cup sweetener*

1/4 cup walnuts

1/4 cup chopped

INSTRUCTIONS

1. Line square baking dish with parchment paper.
2. To make nut butter, process 3/4 cup almonds and 1/2 cup hazelnuts in food processor or bullet blender. Blend until fairly smooth. Add coconut oil to thin if necessary.

3. Chop remaining walnuts and hazelnuts. Add to small bowl with nut butters, cocoa powder, remaining oil, and sweetener and mix well.
4. Spread mixture into parchment lined baking dish and refrigerate for about 2 - 3 hours.
5. Slice and serve chilled or room temperature.

raw honey, agave nectar or maple syrup. Granulated sugar can be used instead. See note for tips on substituting dry sweetener for liquid.

Gluten-Free Dessert Pizza

Prep Time: 15 minutes*

Cook Time: 20 minutes

Servings: 8

Pizza is just another name for pie—and this extra-fruity, thin-crust specialty really delivers. With a layer of lovely vanilla-scented topping and a medley of dried fruits you'll see how truly sophisticated pizza has become.

INGREDIENTS

Crust

1 medium sweet potato

1 cup almond flour

2 eggs

1/4 cup tapioca flour

1 1/2 teaspoon baking powder

1 teaspoon ground cinnamon

1 teaspoon salt

Topping

13 oz (1 can) full-fat coconut milk

2 egg yolks

1 tablespoon tapioca powder

Juice of lemon half

Zest if lemon half

1 teaspoon vanilla

4 dried figs

1/4 cup dried apricots

1/4 cup dried cranberries

1/3 cup dried cherries

INSTRUCTIONS

1. Preheat oven to 350 degrees F. Bring medium pot of lightly salted water to a boil. Cover sheet pan with parchment paper, baking mat, or aluminum foil coated with coconut oil.

2. Peel and dice sweet potato. Add sweet potato and figs to pot and boil 5 - 10 minutes, or until soft.

3. While potatoes boil, heat small pot over medium heat. Add coconut milk, egg yolks, 1 tablespoon tapioca flour, juice and zest of half a lemon. Stir until thickened, about 5 - 10 minutes. Remove from heat and set aside.

4. Drain sweet potatoes and figs in colander. Set figs aside to cool. Add sweet potatoes to medium mixing bowl and mash with hand mixer or whisk. Add 2 eggs and beat well. Then mix in, almond flour, tapioca flour, baking powder, cinnamon and salt with wooden spoon to form dough.

5. Place dough on sheet pan and cover with parchment sheet. Press into round disc with palms, then flatten with rolling pin if desired. Remove top parchment sheet.

6. Bake crust for 20 minutes until center is firm and edges are lightly browned.

7. Chop softened figs and apricots.

8. Carefully remove crust and turn oven to broil. Evenly spread coconut lemon sauce over crust and sprinkle with dried fruit.

9. Return pizza to oven and broil for 2 minutes, just to heat toppings.

10. Remove pizza from oven. Slice and serve warm.

stevia, raw honey or agave nectar. Granulated sugar or stevia can be used instead. See note for tips on substituting dry sweetener for liquid.

Un-Mascarponed Tiramisu

Prep Time: 20 minutes*

Cook Time: 10 minutes

Servings: 8

You may know that tiramisu is Italian slang for an afternoon pick-me-up. With its little kick from the espresso, this afternoon favorite will get you through a long day in style. You will be amazed by the caramel cream that replaces the traditional mascarpone cheese. Heavenly.

INGREDIENTS

Lady Fingers

1/3 cup coconut flour

3 tablespoons arrowroot powder

4 eggs

1/4 cup sweetener**

1/2 teaspoon baking powder

1/2 teaspoon vanilla

2 tablespoons instant espresso (or instant coffee)

3/4 cup water

2 tablespoons cocoa powder

Cashew Mascarpone

2 cups cashews

2 tablespoons sweetener**

1 teaspoon lemon juice

1 teaspoon vanilla

Water

INSTRUCTIONS

1. *Soak 2 cups cashews in water overnight. Drain and rinse.
2. Preheat oven to 400 degrees F. Line two sheet pans with parchment paper. Fit pastry bag with 1/2 inch round tube, or cut 1/4 inch corner off sturdy kitchen storage bag (like Ziploc®).
3. Beat egg yolks, 1/4 cup sweetener and 1/2 teaspoon vanilla until thick and pale.
4. In separate bowl beat egg whites to stiff peaks with hand mixer or whisk in medium bowl. Fold half of egg whites into egg yolk mixture. Then sift in coconut flour, arrowroot powder and baking powder. Fold in remaining egg whites.
5. Scoop batter into pastry bag or storage bag. Place in tall wide contain and fold open end of bag over edge of container for greater ease.
6. Pipe 5 inch lady fingers onto parchment lined sheet pans about 2 inches apart. Bake for 8 minutes.
7. Remove cookies from oven and transfer full parchment sheet onto wire rack to cool completely. Do not try to remove warm cookies from parchment.
8. Process soaked cashews in food processor or bullet blender with sweetener, lemon juice, vanilla, and just enough water to smooth.
9. Bring 3/4 cup water just under a boil. Dissolve instant espresso or coffee in water and add to shallow dish.

10. Remove cooled lady fingers form parchment. Dip and roll each cookie in espresso, then arrange in single layer in glass baking dish. Cut cookies to fit into tight layer.

11. Dollop and spread on half of *Cashew Mascarpone*. Then add another layer of espresso dipped lady fingers. Top with last half of *Cashew Mascarpone* and sift on cocoa powder.

12. *Refrigerate at least 30 - 60 minutes.

13. Slice and serve chilled.

*stevia, raw honey or agave nectar. Granulated sugar or stevia can be used instead. See note for tips on substituting dry sweetener for liquid.

Mixed Berry Trifle

Prep Time: 10 minutes

Cook Time: 25 minutes

Servings: 12

Trifle is perfect all year 'round. Whether the star of a holiday buffet, the crowning jewel at a summer garden party, or bursting with spring's beauty at a Mother's Day tea, it is never out of place. Layers of sweet berries, coconut cream, and delicate almond sponge, all topped with a lovely veil of pale green pistachios—it really doesn't get much better than that.

INGREDIENTS

Cake

1 cup almond flour

1 cup coconut flour

3/4 cup coconut milk

4 eggs

1/2 cup sweetener*

1/2 cup coconut or other cooking oil

2 tablespoons vanilla

2 teaspoons baking soda

Filling

1 cup coconut cream

2 tablespoons sweetener*

1 cup strawberries

1/2 cup blueberries

1/2 cup raspberries

1/2 cup blackberries

Juice of orange half

Juice of lemon half

Zest of orange half

Zest of lemon half

1/4 cup pistachios

INSTRUCTIONS

1. Preheat oven to 350 degrees F. Line muffin pan with paper liner or coat with oil.
2. In large mixing bowl, beat eggs and coconut milk until light and airy. Beat in sweetener, oil and vanilla.
3. Sift in almond flour, coconut flour and baking soda. Mix until well combined.
4. Use ice cream scoop or spoon to scoop batter into muffin pan. Fill each cup 1/2 - 2/3 full with batter.
5. Bake in for about 15 minutes, until firm but springy in the center.
6. Remove cupcakes from oven and turn out onto wire rack or plate. Allow to cool for about 10 minutes and remove paper liners.
7. Dice strawberries and add to medium bowl with blueberries, raspberries, blackberries, lemon and orange zests and juices. Toss to combine.
8. In small bowl, mix coconut cream with 2 tablespoon sweetener.
9. Slice cupcake in half to create top and bottom. Dollop coconut cream onto bottom half, then top with a spoonful of fruit. Drain juice from spoon before adding to cake.

10. Place cupcake top on top of fruit. Press down slightly. Add another dollop of coconut cream and another spoonful of fruit. Repeat with remaining cupcakes.
11. Serve room temperature. Or chill for 30 minutes and serve.

NOTE: Bake cake in 3 round cake pans for 20 minutes, then layer with cream and berries and stack for **Mixed Berry Trifle Cake**.

stevia, raw honey or agave nectar. Granulated sugar or stevia can be used instead. See note for tips on substituting dry sweetener for liquid.

Date Cookies

Prep Time: 10 minutes

Cook Time: 15 minutes

Servings: 12

These will remind you of your favorite packaged snack bars—wrap up couple and take them with you when you're on the go. A great, quick-and-easy, alternative to packaged products. Add dried fruit, chocolate bits, or some nuts or seeds to up the wow factor.

INGREDIENTS

1 1/2 cups almond flour

1 cup coconut flour

1/2 cup sweetener*

5 dried pitted dates

1 egg

2 teaspoons coconut or other cooking oil

1 teaspoon vanilla

1/2 teaspoon baking soda

Pinch salt

Water

INSTRUCTIONS

1. Preheat oven to 350 degrees F. Line sheet pan with parchment paper. Bring small pot of water to boil. Add dates and boil for about 5 - 8 minutes, until softened.

2. Add dates to food processor or bullet blender and process until smooth. Add leftover water if necessary.

3. Add sweetener, egg, oil and vanilla to dates and process until smooth.

4. Add date mixture to medium bowl. Sift in almond flour, coconut flour baking soda and salt. Beat with hand mixer until combined and smooth, about 5 minutes.

5. Roll dough into a log about 3 inches in diameter. Slice into 1/4 inch thick disks.

6. Place disks on sheet pan and bake for about 8 - 10 minutes.

7. Remove form oven and cool for a few minutes.

8. Serve warm or room temperature.

stevia, raw honey or agave nectar. Granulated sugar or stevia can be used instead. See note for tips on substituting dry sweetener for liquid.

Carrot Cake Cookies

Prep Time: 10 minutes

Cook Time: 20 minutes

Servings: 12

Carrot cake always seems like the more virtuous dessert choice. Indeed, it is packed with high-energy, nutrient-rich foods in spite of its cakey nature. This one is no different in that regard. But we've left out the wheat and dairy that makes it a no-no on a GF diet. For an indulgent choice that's both delicious and nutritious, skip the chocolate, wheat, and dairy, and make mine carrot!

INGREDIENTS

2 cups almond meal

4 large carrots (2 cups shredded)

3 eggs

1/4 cup coconut or other cooking oil

1/3 cup unsweetened applesauce

1/2 cup coconut flakes

1/4 cup pitted dates

2 teaspoons vanilla

2 teaspoons ground cinnamon

1 teaspoon ground nutmeg

1 teaspoon ground ginger

INSTRUCTIONS

1. Preheat your oven to 350 Degrees F. Line sheet pan with parchment sheet or coat lightly with oil.

2. Grate carrots, or process in food processor or bullet blender until finely chopped. Add to medium bowl.

3. Add eggs, oil, applesauce and dates to food processor or bullet blender. Process until thick, slightly chunky mixture forms. Pour into carrots.

4. Sift in almond meal. Then add spices and vanilla. Mix well with a wooden spoon. Stir in coconut.

5. Form 12 round balls and evenly space on sheet pan. Flatten balls with hand.

6. Bake about 20 minutes, or until firm and golden brown.

7. Remove from oven and allow to cool about 5 minutes.

8. Serve warm or room temperature.

stevia, raw honey or agave nectar. Granulated sugar or stevia can be used instead. See note for tips on substituting dry sweetener for liquid.

Chocolate Almond Biscotti

Prep Time: 15 minutes

Cook Time: 35* minutes

Servings: 6

Biscotti are "twice-baked" cookies with a pleasantly dry and crunchy texture. Neither too sweet, nor too rich, they are just about perfect dipped into coffee for breakfast as the Europeans do, or for an afternoon snack that won't ruin you for dinner. But they are also marvelous with a glass of red wine for a sophisticated evening treat. Be sure to keep plenty on hand for all those moments when you're feeling peckish.

INGREDIENTS

1 cup almond flour

1/2 cup coconut flour

1/2 cup sweetener*

1/3 cup almonds

2 tablespoons cocoa powder

1 teaspoon vanilla

1/2 teaspoon baking soda

1/4 teaspoon salt

INSTRUCTIONS

1. Preheat oven to 350 degrees F. Line sheet pan with parchment paper. Heat medium pan over medium heat.

2. Add almonds to hot dry pan and toast for about 5 minutes, until aromatic. Stir frequently. Remove from heat and set aside.

3. In medium mixing bowl, blend almond flour, coconut flour, cocoa powder, baking soda and salt with hand mixer or whisk.

4. Beat in sweetener and vanilla until well combined and thick, sticky dough forms. Mix in toasted almonds with wooden spoon.

5. Form dough into flattened, uniform mound about 1 inch thick on sheet pan. Pat down mound to keep any almonds from sticking out.

6. Bake for about 15 minutes . Remove and allow to cool for about 15 minutes.

7. Use a very sharp serrated knife to carefully cut biscotti log into 1/2 - 2/3 inch slices. Hold onto the mound and cut on a diagonal. If it becomes crumbly, stick it back together.

8. Lace slice on sides and return to oven for 15 minutes.

9. Try to cut so that you're holding on to the edges of the log to keep it from crumbling. If parts come apart, you can stick them back together as the mixture is still kind of sticky.

10. Lay the biscotti flat and return to oven for 15 minutes.

11. *Turn oven off and leave oven door open a crack. Allow the biscotti to cool and dry for at least 2 hours.

12. Serve room temperature.

*stevia, raw honey or agave nectar. Granulated sugar or stevia can be used instead. See note for tips on substituting dry sweetener for liquid.

Dairy Free Chocolate Mousse

Prep Time: 5 minutes

Cook Time: 5 minutes

Servings: 2

For so many of us on a GF regimen, dairy products are just as bad for us, and just as off-limits. Heavy cream is an essential part of many mousse recipes, but a forbidden part of many of our diets. This incredible mock chocolate mousse will satisfy the craving for that cool, creamy, classic. When you remember that the avocado is a fruit, it might seem a bit less strange! This mistress-of-disguise is simply the smoothest, richest, most chocolaty mousse you can make. You won't wonder where the cream is, but why you don't taste the avocado.

INGREDIENTS

1 3/4 cups (about 2 cans) full-fat coconut milk

1 avocado

1/3 cup sweetener*

2 tablespoons cocoa powder

1 teaspoon vanilla

Handful cacao nibs or chapped nuts (optional)

INSTRUCTIONS

1. Process coconut milk, sweetener, cacao powder and vanilla in food processor or bullet blender until well combined.
2. Slice avocado in half and pit. Scoop flesh into mixture. Process until thick and creamy.

3. Stir in *optional* cacao nibs, nuts, etc.
4. Pour into ramekins or dessert cups and serve immediately. Or refrigerate for 1 hour to thicken.
5. Serve room temperature or chilled.

* raw honey, agave nectar or maple syrup. Granulated sugar can be used instead. See note for tips on substituting dry sweetener for liquid.

.

Old Fashioned Vanilla Pudding

Prep Time: 5 minutes

Cook Time: 10 minutes

Servings: 2

Remember the simple things in life? Vanilla Pudding may seem a bit doughty, but with its simple, basic, and wholesome ingredients, it is the essence of all things good.

INGREDIENTS

13 oz (1 can) coconut milk

2 yolks

3 tablespoons sweetener*

2 tablespoons cacao butter

1 tablespoon vanilla

INSTRUCTIONS

1. Add coconut milk, sweetener and cacao butter to small pot and place over medium heat. Bring to a simmer, stirring periodically. Add vanilla.

2. In small mixing bowl, whisk 1 tablespoon hot coconut milk into egg yolks. Add second tablespoon. Slowly whisk in 1/4 cup of hot liquid, then add yolk mixture back to hot coconut milk.

3. Whisk custard constantly until thickened, about 5 minutes. Do not let pudding burn.

4. Pour hot pudding into ramekins or dessert cups and refrigerate at least 1 hour.
5. Once chilled, serve immediately. Or remove from fridge, and allow to warm up about 10 minutes and serve room temperature.

raw honey or agave nectar. Granulated sugar can be used instead. See note for tips on substituting dry sweetener for liquid.

Frozen Chocolate Cherry Custard

Prep Time: 15* minutes

Cook Time: 20 minutes

Servings: 4

You might call this splendid creation "da *bombe*!" Based on those frozen ice cream orbs, this fruit filled dessert makes a spectacular appearance at any affair. Make sure you've given your ice cream maker canister a good twenty-four hours in the freezer before you begin. I like to store mine—washed, thoroughly dried, and wrapped in a plastic bag—in the freezer at all times so that I'm always ready when it's time to drop the (ice cream) bomb.

INGREDIENTS

13 oz (1 can) full-fat coconut milk

3 oz water

5 egg yolks

1/4 cup sweetener*

1/2 cup pitted cherries

3 tablespoons cocoa powder

2 teaspoons vanilla

INSTRUCTIONS

1. *Freeze ice cream maker canister overnight before to make sure it is cold enough.

2. Heat coconut milk and water in medium pan over medium heat.

3. Slice cherries in half and set aside.
4. While milk is warmed, but not hot, whisk in egg yolks, sweetener and vanilla. Blend well.
5. Sift in cocoa powder and continue whisking until thickened, about 5 minutes.
6. Turn on ice cream maker first, then carefully pour in custard as ice cream maker paddle rotates.
7. Add halved cherries as ice cream maker runs.
8. Freeze mixture about 15 - 20 minutes. Then transfer frozen custard to serving dishes.
9. Serve immediately.

stevia, raw honey, agave nectar or maple syrup. Granulated sugar or stevia can be used instead. See note for tips on substituting dry sweetener for liquid.

Ginger Mango Sherbet

Prep Time: 5* minutes

Cook Time: 15 minutes

Servings: 4

This is a truly inspired combination of flavors in this elegant frozen dessert. It will remind you of the tropics as its warm flavors and cold texture along with herbs and spices combine for a sensual island experience. Be sure to strain the mixture before freezing to ensure its satiny smooth feel.

INGREDIENTS

1 cup almond milk

1 cup coconut milk

2 ripe mangos

2 oz fresh ginger juice (about 8 inch bunch ginger root)

Juice of lime half

Zest of lime half

1 teaspoon vanilla

Bunch fresh mint

INSTRUCTIONS

1. *Freeze ice cream maker canister overnight before to make sure it is cold enough.
2. Add whole peeled ginger root to food processor. Or juice ginger and add to medium mixing bowl. Add mint leaves.

3. Slice, pit and peel mangos. Add to food processor or bullet blender with almond milk. Blend or process until smooth, then strain into medium mixing bowl.

4. Add coconut milk, juice and zest of half a lime, and vanilla. Mix well with whisk or hand mixer.

5. Turn on ice cream maker first, then carefully pour in mango mixture as ice cream maker paddle rotates.

6. Freeze for about 15 - 20 minutes. Then transfer frozen custard to serving dishes.

7. Serve immediately.

Sweet Potato Gnocchi

Prep Time: 20 minutes

Cook Time: 10 minutes

Servings: 2

This unusual dish is for when you want to impress! A sophisticated, gourmet-inspired ending for your next gathering. You and your guests will love its rustic elegance and the surprisingly satisfying taste of spicy sweet potato and vanilla-scented coconut cream. A truly unique and memorable finish.

INSTRUCTIONS

Gnocchi

1 large sweet potato

Pinch salt

1 egg

1 - 2 cups almond flour

1 - 2 cups tapioca flour (or arrowroot powder)

2 teaspoons ground cinnamon

1 teaspoon ground nutmeg

Sauce

1/4 cup pecans

1/4 cup sweetener* (or 1/4 cup dried pitted dates)

1/4 cup full-fat coconut milk

1 teaspoon vanilla

INGREDIENTS

1. Bring medium pot of lightly salted water to boil.
2. Peel, dice and boil sweet potatoes for about 5 - 10 minutes, until soft.
3. Drain sweet potatoes in colander and add to medium mixing bowl. Mash with hand mixer or whisk. Beat in egg, salt and spices.
4. Bring medium pot of water to boil.
5. Beat 1/2 cup almond flour into sweet potato mixture. Alternate with 1/2 cup tapioca flour or arrowroot powder until dough you can roll in your hand forms. It will still be wet and slightly sticky.
6. Dust cutting board with a few tablespoons of almond flour and tapioca or arrowroot.
7. Roll a portion of dough into a snake about 1 inch thick. Slice roll into pieces 1/2 - 2/3 inch wide. Repeat with remaining dough.
8. Add gnocchi to boiling water in small batches. Cook until they float. Remove from water with slotted spoon or handled strainer and set aside.
9. Heat small pan over medium heat and add pecans. Toast about 2 minutes, then add coconut milk and vanilla. Stir in sweetener, or diced dates.
10. Add gnocchi to the pan and cook another minute or two.
11. Serve hot.

stevia, raw honey or agave nectar or maple syrup. Granulated sugar or stevia can be used instead. See note for tips on substituting dry sweetener for liquid.